Heroic Struggle

Coping with Chronic Illnesses

Personal Eczema Experiences

Christine Matama

FOUNTAIN PUBLISHERS
www.fountainpublishers.co.ug

Fountain Publishers
P.O. Box 488
Kampala, Uganda
E-mail: sales@fountainpublishers.co.ug
              publishing@fountainpublishers.co.ug
Website: www.fountainpublishers.co.ug

Distributed in Europe and Commonwealth countries
outside Africa by:
African Books Collective Ltd,
P. O. Box 721,
Oxford OX1 9EN, UK.
Tel/Fax: +44(0) 1869 349110
E-mail: orders@africanbookscollective.com
Website: www.africanbookscollective.com

ISBN 978-9970-25-964-9

Author's contacts:
E-mail: christineabwooli@outlook.com
              matamaabwooli@gmail.com
Mobile: +256 775 461217

Dedication

I dedicate this book to my dear parents, Mr Charles and Mrs Mable Musana; Dr and Mrs Sylvester Kugonza and family who motivated me to write this book; Dr Fred Kambugu, my treating physician; Dr and Mrs Geoffrey Kabagambe Rugamba; Dr Mary Kiconco Begumya Ogara; Dr Victor Musiime; Peggy Van Leeuwen of the Pharm Access — Amsterdam; as well as Mulago National Referral Hospital Skin clinic, National Medical Stores (NMS) and Dr Anatoli Kamale of Medical Research Council (MRC) and Uganda Virus Research Institute — Entebbe, who offered comfort and wise counsel; my siblings: Priscilla Namara (Mrs Mwesigwa), Solomon Musinguzi, Rita Kasana, Nelson Akolebirungi, among other siblings and cousins; Agnes Birungi, Lillian Kugonza, Grace Bagonza, Mr and Mrs Moses Kiyamba, Mr and Mrs Titus Musiime, Betty Kemigisa, Cloris Musa Irumba, Jackline Basemera, Sheba N. Kasoma, Thelma Kiwinda and Jacqueline Akite as well as my aunts and uncles who visited me; my relatives and friends for the love you showed me which gave me resilience to face another day and strength to be able to share this story. My classmates at university (2004–2008); discussion group members: Doreen Akugizibwe (RIP), Lawrence Engorat, Angela Baitwabusa, Pastor Tony Ssekyanzi, Dr Richard Mpango, Mrs Marjorie Muhinda, Jamesa Wagwau and Ms Angela Balaba— thank you for the moral support! To Rev. Etienne and the entire Youth Praise and Worship Team at Rwengoma Church of Uganda — Fort Portal, the Charismatic Team from Town Church Fort Portal, and all other religious groups that gave me moral support — I really appreciate all the help!

Contents

Foreword

You are reading a book that will provide an epic illustration of courage and optimism. This valuable information comes in handy for the reader to have an in-depth understanding of the chronic ailments that will aid in strengthening coping mechanisms in disease management by patients and health workers. My impression of Christine Matama, author, is that she has endured a chronic illness — eczema — and she has also exhibited enormous skills in supporting a greater number of chronically ill patients. She has worked at the Joint Clinical Research Centre, under my leadership.

From her experience as a patient of eczema and over eight years of experience in caring for the chronically ill, Christine Matama provides an informed approach to the management of chronic illnesses and highlights some of the most important unresolved challenges.

She then illustrates how imperative it is to explain the diagnosis to the patient early and empower them with more information about the condition that contributes towards the path to healing.

I highly recommend this book because it provides insights into coping with persistent illnesses and will be of benefit to patients, their families, care providers and the community at large.

Peter N. Mugyenyi, MBChB, DCH, FRCPI, FRCPE, ScD
Executive Director, Joint Clinical Research Centre
Kampala – Uganda, 2017

Acknowledgements

I would like to acknowledge the following people for having contributed tremendously towards the success of this book: Prof. Peter N. Mugyenyi for giving this book a foreword; Dr and Mrs Sylvester Kugonza who offered me moral and psychological support and greatly motivated me to write this book; Dr Fred Kambugu of the Kampala Skin Clinic — my treating physician, who treated me and still does treat me unconditionally; Dr and Mrs Geoffrey Kabagambe and Dr Anatoli Kamale who offered me exceptional care; Dr John K. Nsibambi of Osler Skin Clinic and the entire Skin Clinic of Mulago National Referral Hospital; my employers, Joint Clinical Research Centre (JCRC), Dr Cissy Kityo Mutuluuza, Dr Francis Kiweewa of Walter Reed, Dr Elizabeth Kaudha, Dr Mary Kiconco, Dr Beda Senkware, Dr Bernard Ayebazibwe, Nicholas Bwebare and Emmanuel Kanyemibwa of Fountain Publishers, together with George Okot P'Bitek Oloya for proofreading this work.

Disclaimer

This book is not intended to substitute medical advice from physicians. The reader should regularly consult a physician on matters relating to his/her health and mainly about any signs and symptoms that may necessitate diagnosis or medical attention. The information is only meant to supplement knowledge gaps amongst readers and health workers.

The author and publisher advise readers to take full responsibility for their health and safety and know their limits.

Some names and identifying details have been intentionally changed to protect the privacy of individuals.

Chapter One

Setting the Scene

Nostalgic childhood memories

My name is Christine Matama. I was born and grew up in Fort Portal, western Uganda, on the foothills of the legendary Mountains of the Moon, a region graced with cool weather and friendly people. I was skinny and chocolate-brown.

My childhood memories are of a happy period as I grew up with my parents and siblings. Other relatives, such as my cousins, visited often, and we played and shared a lot of childhood fun, stories and folklore.

My growth and development were without event although, according to my mother, I had a poor appetite. My mother would always have trouble feeding me, earning me and my siblings a fair share of slaps during meal times!

When I was five years old, I was taken to school along with my siblings. While at school, we were beaten a little and waking up early was not fun at all. Late coming attracted punishments such as being pinched on the cheeks or hands, caning or picking litter from the compound and sweeping the classroom. The same punishments were administered when we made noise in class or committed other offences. As children however, the pain was shortlived. We played games and laughed. It was then that I discovered that I was an athlete. I was a fast runner and my friends loved to cheer me on. That made me happy! Although I was brought up in an average family, education was a priority for all of us children. We excelled at school and competed as siblings since we followed one another in class. Besides going to school, we were involved in many household chores to the extent that by the age of 15, we knew the basics of washing clothes, cooking and tiding up a home. Miraculously, we excelled at school and soon we were at secondary and then tertiary institutions.

My childhood was full of happiness and joy. We played games such as hide and seek. In the evening, we fetched water from the village stream near our home that ran through my grandparents' land and this stream was believed to have the cleanest water in the entire village. The water contained a lot of minerals, such as calcium, that stained saucepans. Many families fetched water there. All this came to an end when my parents installed a huge water tank at home. Now, rain water was harvested automatically from the roof top. The government of Uganda also introduced boreholes in rural areas for safe water in the mid-90s.

Food was readily available at a low cost because as a family we practised mixed farming. We reared cattle on a farm. We also planted many crops and fruits, mainly for home consumption. We grew foodstuffs including bananas, sweet potatoes, Irish potatoes, cassava, maize, beans, peas, millet, pumpkins, and sugar cane. We also grew tomatoes, avocados, cabbage, passion fruits, paw paws, guavas, mangoes and blackberries — these were my favourite.

We also visited my great grandmother every weekend; she died at the age of 110. She prepared us locally made food such as roasted beans cooked with groundnuts, young pumpkins and their leaves. We rode a wooden bicycle, played with dolls made from banana fibre and built mud and wattle houses where we played.

Birthday celebrations were mostly arranged for me, maybe because I loved partying and everyone in the family seemed interested in my day. I looked effortlessly cool during those parties.

In 2003, I started my long senior six vacation after I sat the Uganda Advanced Certificate of Education examinations. I chose to spend my holiday with my parents in Fort Portal. I have wonderful memories of this time: breakfast in bed sometimes, ample rest and journeys to visit relatives and fantastic places.

In most traditional schools in Uganda (primary and secondary), plaiting hair is almost taboo. School administrations find it time - consuming and the costs involved place a big burden on the students and parents, so most schools prefer to help pupils/ students to do away with their hair. During long vacations, therefore, students like to grow their hair and look nice and this is what I did.

I had never suffered from any disease or had injections apart from during immunisation and when I was injured back in 1997 as I run in the school cross country competitions; I was a good athlete, back then.

A brief dream-come-true and nightmares

I was barely 19 years old when I joined university. This marked the realisation of a dream that would open doors to fulfilling my other dreams. Attaining university education was perceived as one of lifes' highest achievements. However, all this was about to change into a world of frustration and despair!

During my first year at university, I developed pimple-like swellings on the left side of the face. They have probably appeared because I am still a teenager!' I thought. "But why at this late stage of my teenage?" With time I lost my chocolate-brown colour and my tender smooth skin! I had thought that when I got out of the teenage stage I would kiss the pimples goodbye, I was wrong!

No sooner had I come to terms with these teenage symptoms than I was diagnosed with this strange disease — or Eczema-like rash. My immediate reaction was a feeling of frustration about my inability to pursue my university education. All hope for my successful completion of the course was gone. My motivation had been at its highest peak to study and achieve my dreams, but with this diagnosis, my dreams were almost shattered.

However, I had to look for creative ways to help me live to see my dream of completing university. I was supported by several people, among them, Dr and Mrs Sylvester Kugonza, great family friends. They were fascinated by my zeal and determination to accomplish my dreams — and later challenged me to write this book, a book I was deeply worried that no one would bother to read! Besides, I had other priorities such as taking on postgraduate studies.

Soon, the pimples shifted to the right side of my face. Still, I ignored them. But not long afterwards, my scalp was not spared. Whenever I took a bath, my entire body protested with sharp pain. Worried, I rushed to a dermatologist. I knew I was in danger. "Was I living an unhealthy lifestyle? No! Was it just an illness? What could I do to put my skin out of harm's way?" I wondered.

As the years passed, I grieved hopelessly. The illness took a toll on me physically, mentally, emotionally and financially, resulting in feelings of sorrow, grief, anger and stress. I was admitted to hospital frequently, suffered headaches, swelling and feeling pressure from within, poor appetite and generalised body weakness and I was irritable. Available literature was mostly scholarly and described observation from health workers' perspective, yet I needed to hear from fellow patients battling the same disease. It was not until I had a discussion with my doctor that I learnt that what was disturbing me was stress, which is the body's response to a hopeless situation or series of unpleasant events.

My doctor went on to explain that when one is in such a situation, the brain's hypothalamus gland sends a trigger through the nerves and releases chemicals to the adrenal glands that sit on top of the kidneys. Then the adrenal glands release the cortisol hormone, among other chemicals, affecting one's feelings, thoughts and behaviour. If this stress is not dealt with, this will stir up cravings for sugar and fat, thus causing obesity. Stress is also responsible for many other problems such as poor digestion which affects nutrition or brings about loss of appetite. In some cases, this results into weight loss, headache, high blood sugar, high blood pressure, memory loss and lack of sleep. It compromises immunity and raises many other challenges. So, avoiding stress should be one's principle goal.

I learnt through my doctors that there was nothing much I could do about my condition because most triggers of eczema are not easy to identify. In the end, I was not overly concerned about my appearance and this helped me cope very fast. People talked about the spherical scars on my body and others mistakenly referred to them as ringworms. It was within the same scars that fresh reactions occurred, as if they made a trail for easy come-back!

I consumed lots of drugs; antibiotics and antifungal medicines dominated the doctors' treatment options — from tablets to intravenously administered drugs — but the reaction advanced in its most severe form.

I received a number of medications like Mebendazole 400mg, to fight off worms; Cotrimoxazole tabs to fight off chest infections and on the scalp I used medicated shampoos like Nizoral shampoo, Keto-plus and Keto-mark shampoo, with antifungal components.

I also used coal tar shampoo several times, but stopped it later due to its effect of escalating itching. I used Elocom lotions for the scalp; G.V Paint 1% (purple liquid) for the wounds on the body; topical corticosteroid creams and hydrocortisone creams for the skin; Candid B lotions; Cefodox; Aterax; Aphosyl cream; H/C cream; Clobetasol ointment and Cetrizine to help in itching. I also used Prednisolone, and Salbutamol for the treatment of Asthma; tetracycline creams, Fobancort ointment; Griseofluvin; Butenafine hydrochloride cream (fintop cream), Ketoconazole, fucidic Acid-B cream, Mupirocin ointment and a wide range of antibiotics like Amoxicillin-Clavulanic acid tabs; Cloxaciline tabs; Levo Cloxaciline tabs; Cefriaxone; Metronidazole tabs; fragyl; Doxycyline tabs; Benzathine penicillin; Promethazine Hydrochloride tabs; Aminophylline tabs; Erythromycin tabs; Linezolid tabs, Ciprobed flu butane creams; Aminophyillice tabs; Beeto cream, Epimax cream, Ecocort creams for smearing on the skin and Probeta N ointments for the eyes. These were from doctors' prescriptions mostly.

What was clear was that Prednisolone, Cetrizine, antibiotics like Amoxicillin Clavulanic acid tabs (Amoxiclav) and antifungals like Ketoconazole dominated the doctors' treatment options. This was after a culture and sensitivity test was performed on an ear swab that tested and detected Gram-positive cocci with some in pairs sensitive to Augmentin also known as Clavam, Oxacillin, Zinnat and resistant to Gatifloxacin, Cotrimoxazole, Tetracycline and Erythromycin. Culture and sensitivity tests and resistance tests are a must to help doctors make informed decisions on the best medications to give to a patient. Prolonged use of some of these medications result into resistance of germs to these drugs and therefore require culture and sensitivity tests to determine the best medication. Resistance happens when germs change their form and drugs fail to take the desired effect. Just like resistance happens to antiviral drugs, the same happens to antibiotics.

I also had a taste of antihistamines like Fexofen Hydrochloride 120mg (Allegra). These block histamines that cause allergies in the body.

I took these drugs religiously and not just for one or two months, but many months that culminated into years — we are talking of 14 years now!

My wonderful Ugandan friends working in the United Kingdom and others from Amsterdam took the initiative to consult dermatologists for a remedy for me and they came up with an emulsifying ointment (Emollient) that helps keep my skin well hydrated; it emulsifies the skin, giving it its lost glory. My treating doctor was positive about it, and they also suggested Epaderm. However, Epaderm caused a lot of itching and I stopped using it.

I consumed all sorts of herbs and Chinese/Japanese or Asian medicines that are approved as supplements. The most common herb that I used was aloe vera. I showered, drunk and smeared it on my body in vain. Because of my skin's hypersensitivity, itching and the burning sensation, I could hardly use cold water to bathe, so I turned to using lukewarm water. I also resorted to using gentle oils and skin products to moisturise my skin; those without any fragrance or alcohol, otherwise, I risked aggravating the already awful situation. Products that contain alpha hydroxy acids, avobenzone, octinoxate, oxybenzone, glycolic acid and retinol are known irritants and it was difficult to know that they were in certain skin products that I used. I faced difficulty getting the best products. My way out was to use plain vaseline, baby oil, shea butter oil, coconut oil, and olive oil, for my skin and hair.

Episodes of reactions unfolded like some sort of script and this was terrifying. People who saw me had their own recommendations, beliefs and misconceptions for what I should eat or avoid. They recommended different herbal remedies and some desperately brought them home, to see me get well again. When the illness was at its worst, lots of messages kept flowing in from friends and family on whether to or not sunbathe for fear of getting skin cancer, or to bathe cold water or not.

It was disheartening because I wasn't getting any better. The eczema started showing up in places on my body where it had never been before, sneaking up from my legs, to my arms, armpits, neck and finally my back. My physician had at some point asked me for information on previous medications that worked for me. These included steroids, topical creams and antibiotics. He gave me directions on their moderate use. He even pulled out textbooks to enlighten me on the condition and gave me handouts about the condition. I felt empowered to monitor myself on medication.

My physician occasionally requested to see me in the company of his students and on one occasion I overheard the students asking amongst themselves: "What else will be asked about her?" Little did I know that I was being observed as the best candidate for a scholarly activity involving students on the Master's degree in dermatology at Makerere University.

He requested for my consent to be a participant and I accepted because I wanted to play a critical role in bringing a difference in scholarly activities and consequently, new treatments. So he asked them what they thought the disease was. I was very ill. I could hardly walk, with fluid oozing out of the skin and mostly joints. I could hardly stretch my arms and legs, the itchy rash was all over my body and my feet were swollen. When the physician asked the student what they thought the disease was, their responses were: "It is liver cirrhosis," "Tuberculosis (TB) of the skin," "an HIV-related skin condition" and "Psoriasis." Others said it was cancer of the skin while others suggested a skin biopsy. Though I was very ill, I felt at ease with my physician and his students were friendly and humorous.

My fellow students in the counselling class suspected that I had the Human Immunodefiency Virus (HIV) that causes Acquired Immune Deficiency Syndrome (AIDS). They recommended that I get tested. Some counselled me endlessly. Some discriminated against me — I felt out of place. I was baffled when the guy I was dating gave me a cold shoulder! Not long after that, the relationship ended.

The pimple-like rash spread throughout my body aggressively, like army worms on the loose, this time with secondary bacterial infection. My body was covered with pus, a greasy substance and a yellowish fluid oozed out of the skin. I would wash it off in the morning. By day, the body would develop scales and the same rash would be back by evening. Over time, the hair on my scalp waned and the scalp became more sensitive.

Much as loss of hair is a typical sign of lack of Biotin (Vitamin B), this was representative of eczema. As the skin dried up, dandruff-like particles would shed off, covering the entire bed and the bedroom floor. My parents were involved in endless cleaning. They changed my beddings at midnight and in the morning. They washed every day; washing away tiny pieces of my skin that looked like dust, "No wonder the clergy say, 'from dust to dust,'" my mum would exclaim! If you stepped in our house barefoot, you would carry away parts of my skin particles!

My parents often carried me out on a sunny day to sunbathe. I would sleep under the scorching sun, naked, save for a sheet covering me. This was my only enjoyable moment outdoors. The itching and swelling eased, but the inflammation did not go completely. My siblings kept watch to wave away ravenous flies that hovered around me, while my parents tirelessly gave me the cold drinks that I yearned for.

I experienced hot flushes in my stomach and, therefore, required cold drinks. There was barely any skin on my palms, which meant that I could not hold a cup of hot or warm tea. I would be straw-fed when I needed to take warm tea.

Out of despair, prayers became the order of the day. My parents were so terrified that they succumbed to pressure from the village community that the nature of my condition needed the intervention of the Charismatic Prayer Team. My parents hardly slept as they had to support me each night. They would wake up in the wee hours of the night to change my beddings and then they would say a word of prayer and feed me. I endured cold nights that would make me cough. Thankfully, my parents and family were supportive. Relatives and friends kept trickling in to have a "last look" at me while others asked if I had my wits about me, given the number of wounds on my scalp. "Let us go and visit her before she dies. This is no ordinary disease!" relatives lamented.

A lot of money was spent on costly tests and drugs. With no insurance, my healthcare costs soared to close to $1,000 per month, including visiting other specialists like the Ear, Nose and Throat (ENT) clinic. I spent so much money and time visiting numerous doctors, to no avail. I felt I had exhausted all my resources and I needed a different approach.

I was very impatient and wanted to get well immediately. Complete strangers empathised, others offered money, while others in public transport spared me the fees. Others ignored their own pain at the clinic to offer me a seat so that I could see the doctor before I died. Others offered unsolicited information on the likely causative agent as witchcraft. "It's unfortunate you inherited your parents' curse," they commented.

I underwent several clinical tests; kept a food journal and monitored the foods I ate, including avoiding dairy products for three months, under the close supervision of a medical doctor. It was quite difficult to keep a food diary because food allergies could happen even after days. I turned to only light-coloured cotton clothes; I would also wrap cotton wool around my body to keep warm and to absorb the fluid oozing from my skin. I relocated from relatively warm Kampala to relatively cooler Fort Portal, all in vain. The skin got ragged and my lymph nodes got swollen in some unusual areas, like the temple, behind the ears, below and around the neck.

I suffered other health conditions: hypersensitive skin, allergic conjunctivitis (eye inflammation), pneumonia, hay fever, fish allergies, vitamin deficiencies, anaemia and bacterial, viral and fungal infections. I also got blurred vision from inflammation of the eye lids, ear infections, suffered from asthma, skin fungal infections and my nails got deformed with depressions and white patches.

Thoughts of doom invaded and I could not endure the torment anymore. I broke down in anger when my doctor said; "I am perplexed by your condition." My mind went blank and I could not communicate with him anymore. I picked the drugs and went home. While at home I felt that if the best doctor available for me in Uganda was confused, then it was of no use to continue taking the drugs. I then made a firm decision to stop all the medication. It was a dangerous move and the situation could have quickly gotten out of hand. I developed pneumonia that was not treated. I needed to hide, but meeting people was unavoidable and, besides, I also had to go back to university. Itching was the order of the day. I was full of anger and at some point I directed it at some people, especially those who asked about my state. Perhaps some people resented me for causing them pain. I felt that my days were numbered, but I had to cope with my condition. My classmates and friends expressed concern and cared although some of my classmates thought that it was a contagious disease.

My villagemates thought it was witchcraft. My workmates thought it was HIV. My doctors however made the right diagnosis. They educated me, shared information materials with me to read and understand more about the condition, the impact and its nature. Later, as I improved, I completed my studies at university. The spell of death was broken, I was able to escape the fate that haunted me for so long although the painful memories remained. I was eager to start working. To keep my mind off negative and sad thoughts, I started volunteering at a Non Governmental Organisation and later pursued a Master of Science in Public Health to polish my skills.

I have lived to tell the tale. I am not totally healed from eczema, but I see progress. I have learned to cope with a chronic illness, adapting to the illness and living positively. It is an approach that one needs to embrace at all costs. Treating chronic illnesses is a dreadful prospect because most chronic illnesses do not have a complete cure and they are usually costly to manage.

Light at the end of the tunnel

The 25th February, 2008 was an auspicious day in my life. I graduated with a Bachelor's degree in Guidance and Counselling. The day I graduated started with a heavy downpour in all parts of Kampala where the graduation ceremony was going to take place. I woke up very early, eagerly waiting to head to the university. Traffic was bumper-to-bumper. The heavy rains had caused floods. Cars could hardly move, and my family resorted to walking 200 metres to the graduation grounds.

Finally, we were there — smartly dressed, though wet. I was exhausted and yet excited, together with other jubilant graduands, our families, my former nursery teacher who was also a graduand, and other friends who had gathered to witness this academic achievement.

Later after the university function, I hosted my guests to a luncheon. All around Kampala and its outskirts, similar parties were taking place, but mine seemed special in some way. Here I was, a village girl from Fort Portal in the far west Uganda, graduating with a Bachelor's in Guidance and Counselling — having defied all odds, particularly a strange debilitating illness!

Chapter Two

Eczema at a glance

When my skin was under attack, "rough croc skin" is what people called it when talking about me. Eczema was eating away my skin. Eczema is an immunodeficiency disorder/disease. An immunodeficiency disorder occurs when the immune system's ability to fight off infectious diseases and cancers is compromised or completely absent. The immune system is composed of organs in the body and white blood cells. The cells are made in the bone marrow and travel through the bloodstream and lymph nodes. They protect and defend against attacks by "foreign" invaders such as germs, viruses, bacteria and fungi. Antibodies are proteins that are made in response to an infection or immunisation and help fight infections. When the body lacks this ability to fight infections; lacks proteins or the immune system is not functioning properly, then an immunodeficiency condition occurs.

Immunodeficiency is categorised into two: primary (inborn, hereditary or genetic) and secondary.

Primary immunodeficiency disorders — also called primary immune disorders or primary immunodeficiency — weaken the immune system, making it unable to fight off infections.

Examples of primary immunodeficiency include: severe combined immunodeficiency (SCID); X-linked agammaglobulinemia (XLA), and common variable immunodeficiency (CVID). These are characterised by recurrent infections, low antibody levels; for example low immunoglobulin (Ig — IgE, IgD, IgG, IgM and IgA), as well as auto-immune conditions like eczema, psoriasis, vitiligo and rheumatoid arthritis. Auto-immune disorders happen as a result of a violent attack of the body against its own normal tissues and cells. The body fails to differentiate between self and non-self; it makes antibodies that are directed towards the body's own tissues. These are called auto-antibodies. The auto-antibodies attack the normal cells and tissues by mistake, causing auto-immune diseases or chronic infections.

Secondary (acquired) immunodeficiency happens when one's body gets into contact with an outside infection or agents, for example, chemotherapy, other drugs used during organ transplants, mercury, environment toxins, pesticides, HIV, cancers or viral hepatitis, among others. These conditions hinder the body's ability to protect itself against diseases and the individual suffers chronic diseases or recurrent infections. A normal immune system produces proteins called antibodies which are known as immunoglobulin and which protect the body from infections. In primary immunodeficiency, the body produces "bad" or auto-antibodies which then cause auto-immune diseases that attack normal cells and tissues of the body.

Immunoglobulin A (Ig A) is mostly found in the mucus membranes; Immunoglobulin G (Ig G) is found abundantly in all body fluids and protects against bacteria and viruses while Immunoglobulin M (Ig M), which is the first anti-body to appear when the body is fighting off new infections is found in blood and lymph. Immunoglobulin E (Ig E) is associated mainly with allergic reaction and found in mucus, lungs and skin while Immunoglobulin D (Ig D) exists in small amounts in the body and is not well understood.

Figure 1.1 Types of immunodeficiency

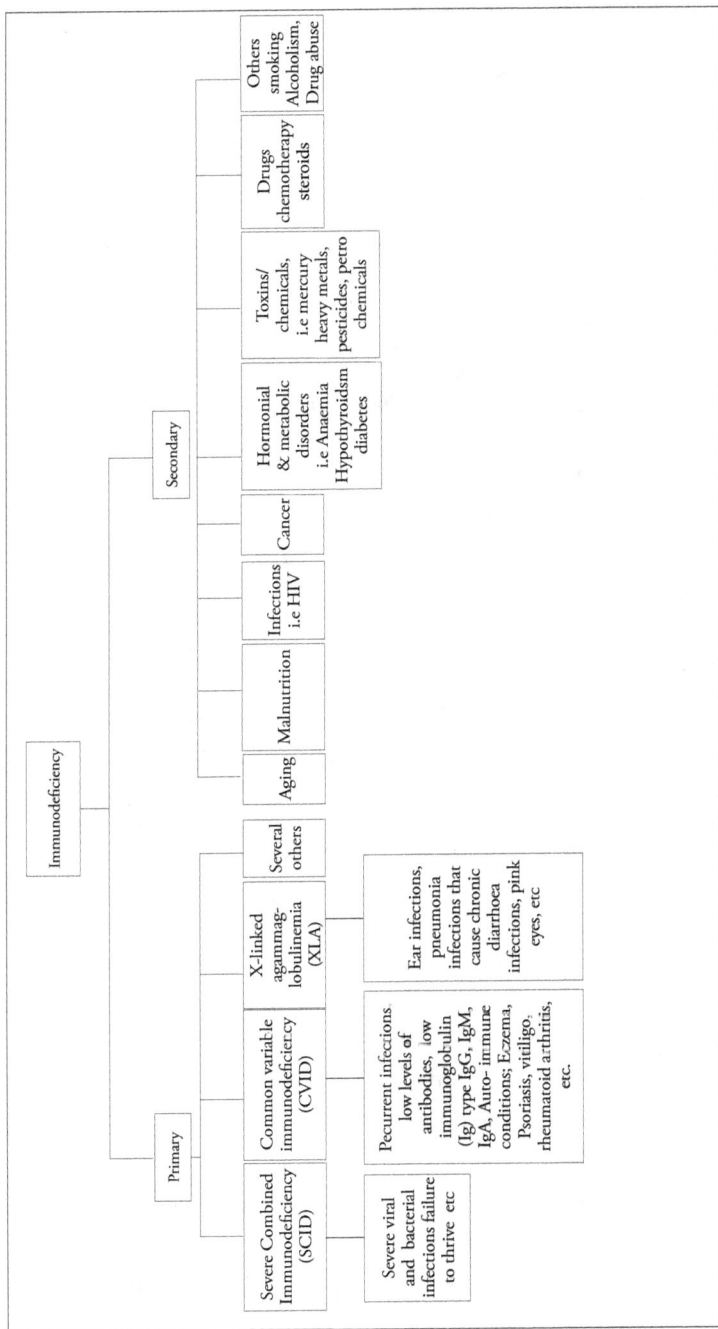

Immunodeficiency

Primary
- Severe Combined Immunodeficiency (SCID)
  - Severe viral and bacterial infections failure to thrive etc
- Common variable immunodeficiency (CVID)
  - Pecurrent infections. low levels of antibodies, low immunoglobulin (Ig) type IgG, IgM, IgA, Auto-immune conditions; Eczema, Psoriasis, vitiligo. rheumatoid arthritis, etc.
- X-linked agammaglobulinemia (XLA)
  - Ear infections, pneumonia infections that cause chronic diarrhoea infections, pink eyes, etc
- Several others

Secondary
- Aging
- Malnutrition
- Infections i.e HIV
- Cancer
- Hormonial & metabolic disorders i.e Anaemia Hypothyroidsm diabetes
- Toxins/ chemicals, i.e mercury heavy metals, pesticides, petro chemicals
- Drugs chemotherapy steroids
- Others smoking Alcoholism, Drug abuse

When one has an auto-immune condition, their immune system attacks normal cells, and so, they are prone to various infections, such as bacterial, fungal and other illnesses. In some people, these auto-antibodies do no harm. Eczema is a skin disease that is a result of an auto-immune condition that is common in primary immunodeficiency disorders, although it can also affect people with a normal immune system.

In my case, low or a deficiency of Immunoglobulin G (Ig G) predisposed me to chronic eczema that left me with a swollen and a deformed body. Eczema is chronic in a sense that it keeps recurring and is persistent for a long time, without completely getting healed. My doctor prescribed Immunoglobulin G (Gammaquin injvlst) for one year which was bought in Germany at £233.35, in 2007.

Eczema, also known as dermatitis, is a skin condition that brings about itching and inflammation. It is characterised by red, fluid-filled blisters. The skin is itchy, dries in patches, often cracks, becomes rough and then thickens. It affects those areas rich in sebaceous glands (substances found in the skin that secrete oily or waxy matter called sebum to lubricate the skin or hair). These areas include the face, behind the ears, the scalp, the back, the joints and the centre of the chest, among others. Where there is itching, scratching follows and the skin's barrier is weakened. This causes greasy oozing of liquid from the affected areas and secondary bacterial infection may occur, causing pus to form in the affected areas. Eczema is classified in many ways or forms:

Atopic eczema is where the skin gets inflamed and itchy. It is sometimes referred to as infantile or childhood eczema. It is caused by abnormality in the functioning of the immune system. When it flares up, it makes the skin red and sore. It may calm down later and the skin becomes dry and itchy. The commonly affected body parts include the face, back, neck, back of knees, front of elbows and the wrist. It affects mostly children, even though older people also get affected.

Contact eczema is sometimes referred to as contact allergic dermatitis or irritant contact eczema. Usually the individual is affected on the part of the body that is in contact with the irritants, for example, detergents, wall paint, poison, skin care products, tobacco smoke, nickel found in jewellery, certain rough clothing, hair styling additions, flowers or perfumes. The individual's skin may appear red and the person experiences burning. It also gets itchy. Severity depends on frequent contact with irritants. It usually affects the hands and face, but other parts of the skin can get affected.

Nummular or discoid eczema affects the skin in circular or coin-shaped patches which are extremely itchy and scaly. They normally start from the legs then the arms, buttocks and the back. The patches ooze and become itchy and crusted. It is common in elderly men.

Seborrheic eczema is the type that affects the scalp and sometimes other parts of the skin. Its cause is unknown, but it is characterised by yellowish, oily, scaly patches and immense itching of the affected areas and other parts of the skin that have grease glands. It is exasperated by over-growth of *Malassezia* yeast on the skin and weather conditions (too much cold or heat). Oily skin and stress may worsen the situation.

Neurodermatitis, also known as Lichen simplex chronicus, occurs after a scratch or when an insect bite has been scratched. The affected area becomes intensely irritated through scratching and it becomes scaly and thick. It is similar to contact eczema and usually women are more affected than men.

Dyshidrotic eczema is when the soles and palms get affected. They get blisters that burst open, followed by itchless, scaling and and burning sensation.

Herpeticum eczema is associated with the herpes simplex virus and usually people with atopic eczema are affected. It can cause high temperatures and swelling of the lymph glands. It is treated with antiviral drugs.

Stasis dermatitis usually affects the legs and is associated with blood circulation where the valves in the veins have been compromised. This causes fluid build-up and consequent blistering. Victims experience itchy skin and oozing of skin lesions. It affects mostly people in old age.

Eczema affects people of all ages and ethnicity. It can be exasperated by stress and except for Herpeticum eczema, it is non-contagious or non-infectious. It has nothing to do with not bathing properly. It is tough to deal with and with frequent flare-ups, it is difficult to maintain a positive outlook. Itching is the order of the day and it is worse at nights. I spent sleepless nights scratching. Conducting blood tests was difficult because of the swollen and flared-up skin.

In my case, Contact eczema made my skin hypersensitive to irritants such as dyes, pollen, fabrics, soaps, animal fur, dust and fragrances/perfumes, among others. In the process, the skin got secondary bacterial infections and the entire body was affected. The environmental factors played a big role in stimulating these reactions and, therefore, it became difficult to distinguish it from other types of eczema (Atopic, Seborrheic and Nummular) and other skin disorders.

It required the services of a dermatologist to distinguish eczema from other forms of skin disorders like psoriasis. An eczema patient gets raised patches which leak fluid and bumps that cause intense itching, mostly at night. They get dry, become flaky or peel off when scratched. On the other hand, psoriasis is diagnosed when skin cells go through their life cycle more quickly than normal — approximately 3 to 4 days, yet the normal period for a cell to regenerate takes one month — this results in patches of thick, scaly and silvery dead cells that pile up on the skin, usually on the elbows and knees, but they can also appear anywhere and cause mild itching. The two conditions are treated the same way and seborrheic eczema tends to be similar to psoriasis.

According to the Dermatological Society (2012), eczema in the United States of America affects between 3 and 5 per cent of the population, both children and adults, but it tends to lessen with age. It attacks areas of the body that are rich with sebaceous glands. It is still not yet clearly understood, but it is believed that the yeast called *Malassezia ovale* (M. ovale), previously known as *Pityrosporum ovale*, which induces scaling and inflammation (irritation, swelling, tenderness), is commonly found on our skins and hydrolyses the sebum that releases a mixture of saturated and unsaturated fatty acids. Then, the fatty acids are taken up by the yeast and unsaturated fatty acids remain and breach the barrier which protects the skin, therefore causing inflammation.

When it comes to avoiding the triggers that cause a reaction to certain conditions, many people may not appreciate what one is going through. Some tend to think that one is looking for attention.

Appearance and distribution on the hair, scalp and body

Eczema is not known locally, let alone having a local name, but it usually appears on the skin, scalp, face and eyebrows. Sometimes, one may get conjunctivitis (inflammation of eyes), swollen or inflamed lips, nose folds or mucus discharge from the nose (not necessarily a cold). It may appear on nose ridges, ear folds and in the ear canal, joint folds, nails, palms, the chest, stomach and upper back or buttocks, which become red. Sometimes it manifests as greyish scaly patches that flake or peel off, and these are usually greasy, oily and itchy.

This results into an itchy scalp and hair loss with thick crusts forming dandruff in the hair or on the body. This may result into raised or swollen skin on the eyebrows and eyes. One may get blurred vision and depressions on the nails. These symptoms may be escalated by fungal or bacterial infections, staphylococcus aureus commonly known as staph germs which become recurrent. The dryness of the skin can also result in painful cracking.

Likely aetiology of Eczema

It is not clear what the cause of Eczema is. It is presumed to be triggered by a genetic predisposition to inheriting the illness, hormonal changes, urbanisation characterised by poor housing conditions, environmental degradation and climate change. A slight change or sudden drop in temperature; changes in lifestyles; exposure to chemicals and other hazardous substances, through touching, eating, drinking and breathing; stress, poverty (leading to lack of access to essential needs) and pollution — all can trigger eczema. In addition, a weakened immune system, smoking or secondary smoking, alcohol consumption, exposure to plastics and pesticides, pollen from flowers, dust, cold weather, animal dander, powdered soaps, soaps with fragrance, walls with moulds and rugs in the house can be blamed for stimulating the condition. Medical practitioners still do not know the likely aetiology of this condition, making it difficult to treat and manage. No specific site on the web or research claims to have information on the likely causative agent.

Eczema is hard to treat and more so to diagnose since it is eerily similar to other skin disorders such as Lupus, Psoriasis, Acne vulgaris, rosacea and allergies. However, it affects the face, eyebrows, upper body and the groin area. To make a diagnosis, a doctor performs a physical examination and sometimes a skin biopsy may be performed to determine what condition it is.

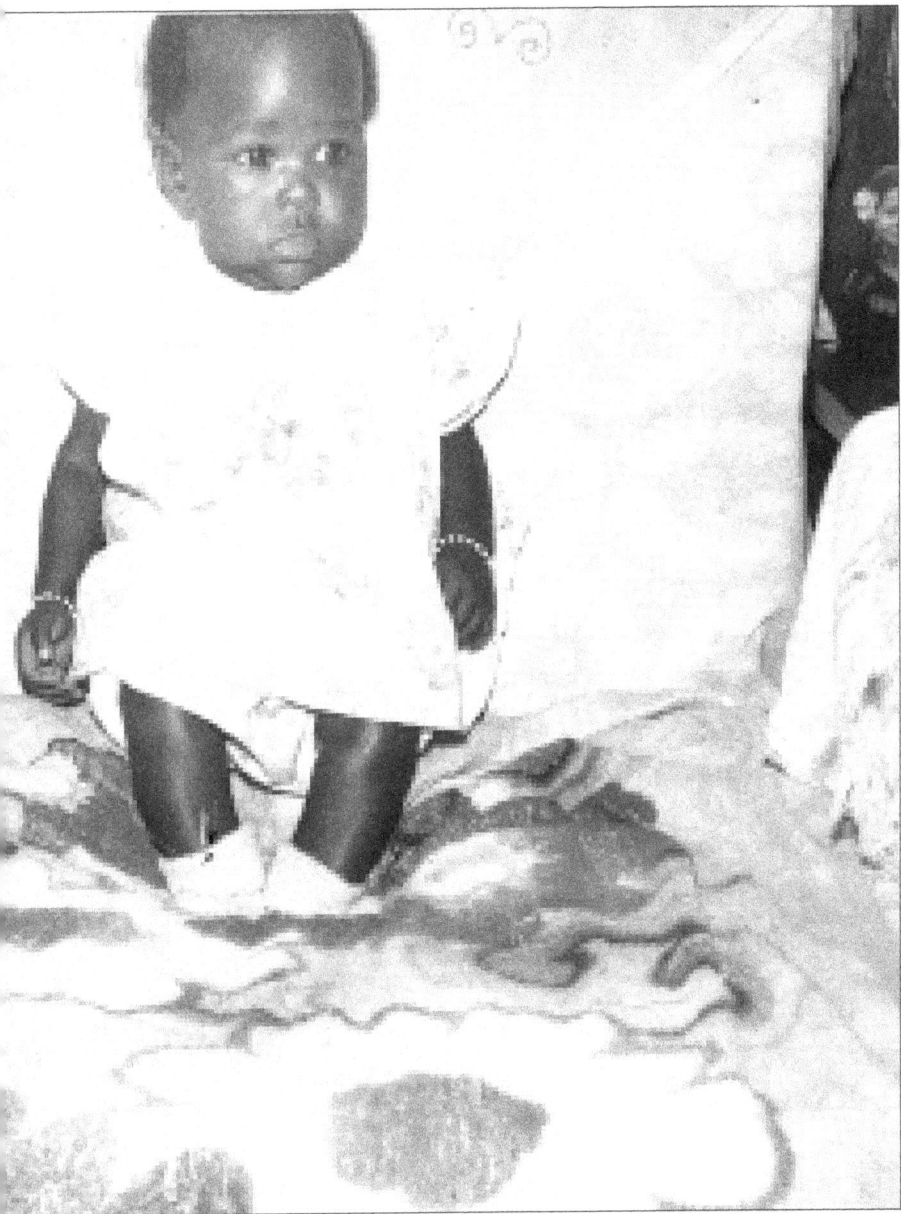

Above: Christine as a baby

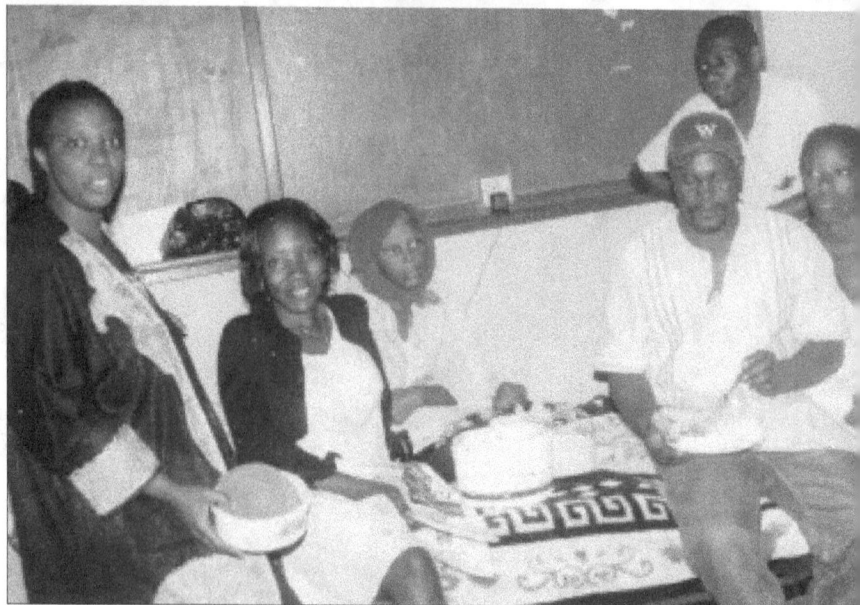

Above: Christine, her siblings and Mum at Mulago National Referral Hospital, 2006

Below: The writer (centre) — a typical Eczema patient — with visible reactions on the scalp (folliculitis). With her, is her younger sister and mother in 2007. Folliculitis is an inflammation of the hair follicles; it is often caused by a bacterial or fungal infection.

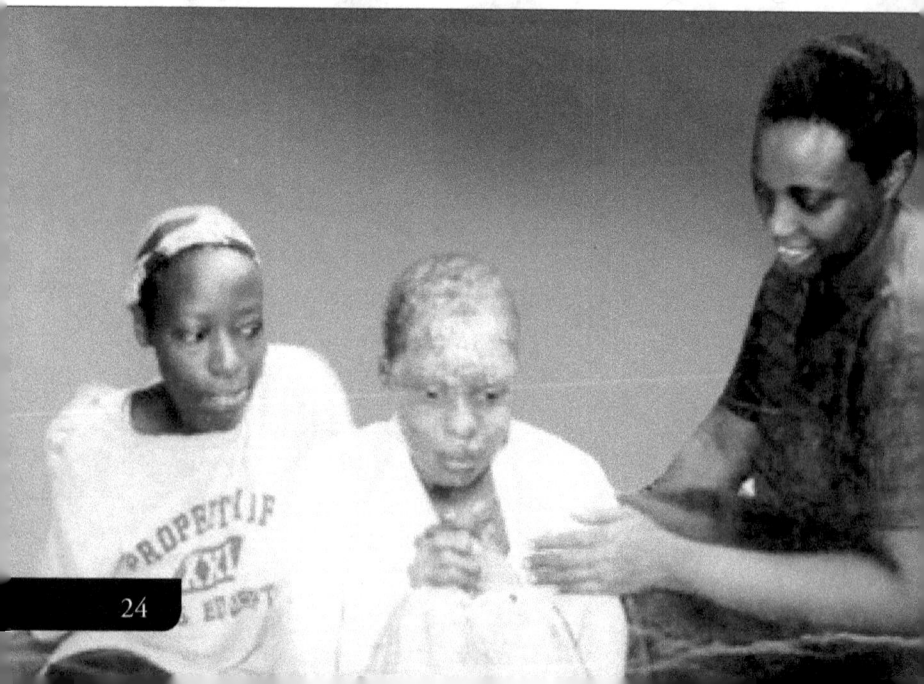

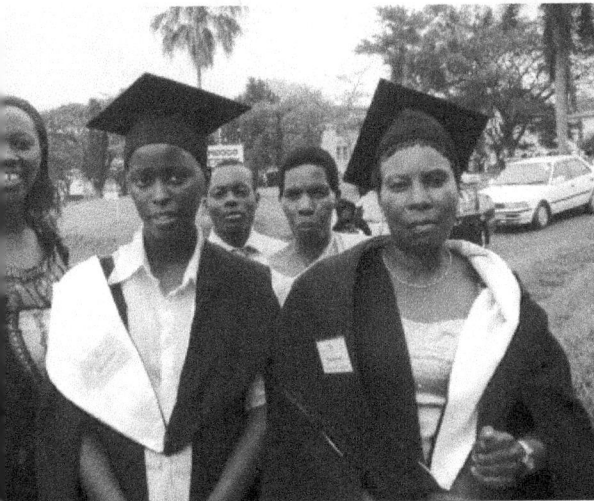

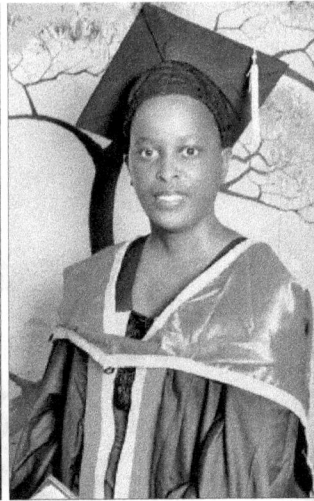

Above left: Christine with her mum (left) and her nursery school teacher (right). Christine and her teacher graduated at the same time (undergraduate degree), February 2008

Above right: Christine on her graduation with a Master of Science in Public Health, 2015

Left: Christine with her parents and siblings on her graduation with a (bachelor's degree), 2008

Below: Christine on her graduation (Bachelor's degree), her mum, Mrs Kugonza, Dr Kugonza and her dad, 2008

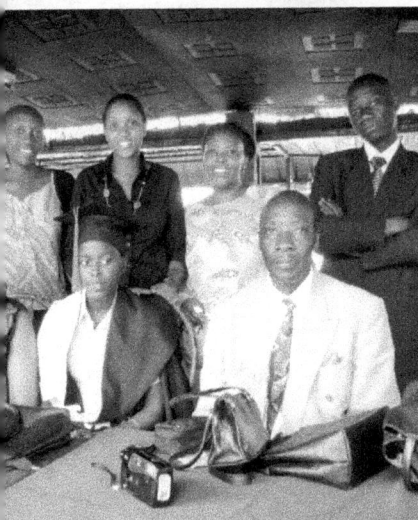

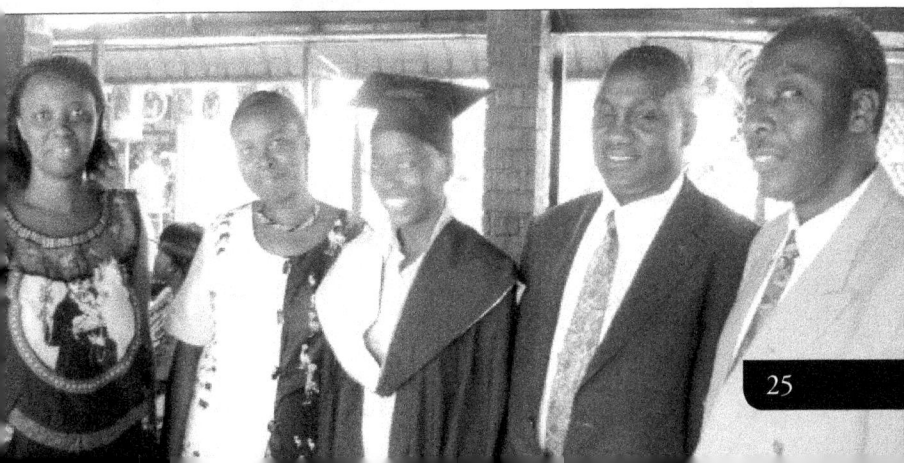

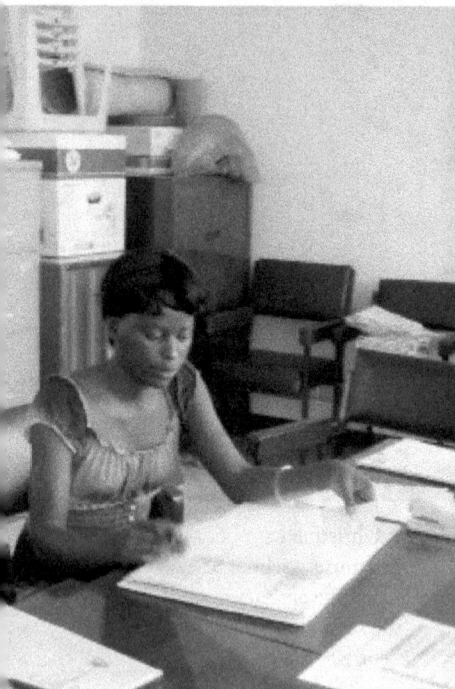

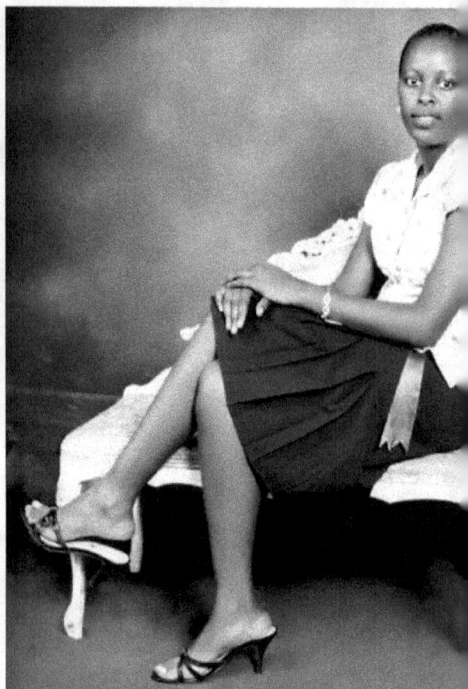

Above left: Christine monitoring, Pharm Access African Studies to Evaluate HIV drug Resistance – Monitoring (PASER-M) Research at Coast Province General Hospital in Mombasa, 2008

Above right: Christine in 2009

Below: Christine gives guidance to a patient living with a chronic illness, 2012

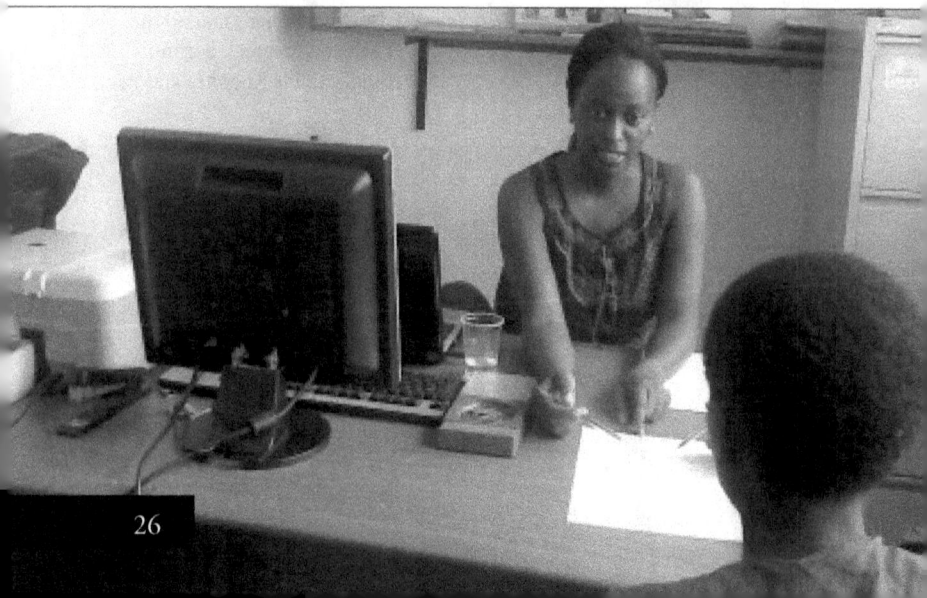

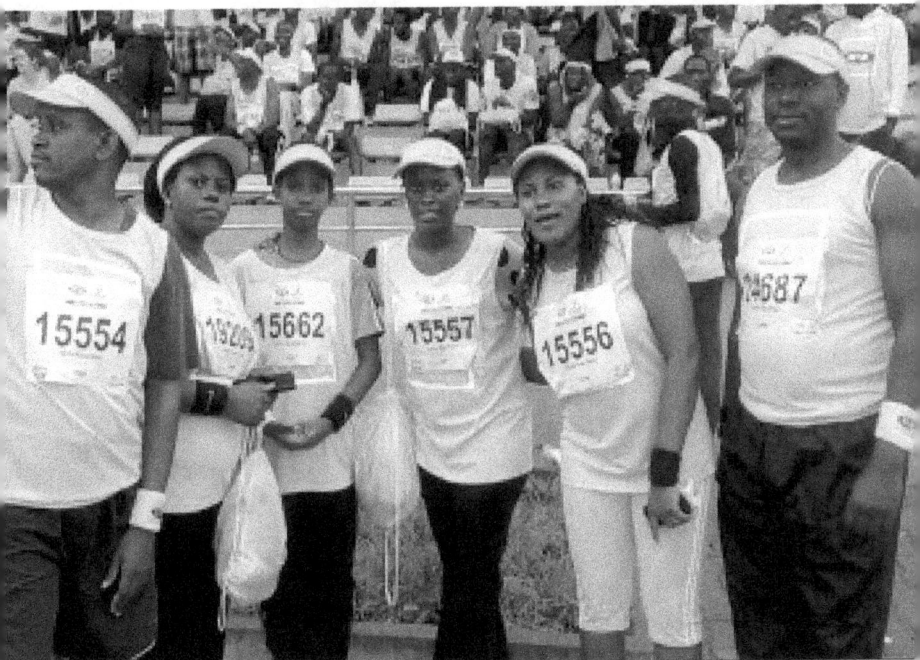

Above: Christine (third from right) with friends after a charity run organised by MTN Uganda, 2014

Below left: Christine (third from right), Martin Asingwire and Mrs Grace Asingwire at Namboole National Stadium for a Uganda Cranes match

Below right: Christine and her workmates participated in the Malaika School run, 2016. Proceeds went to palliative care

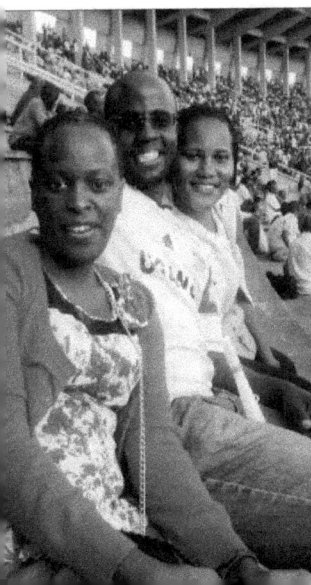

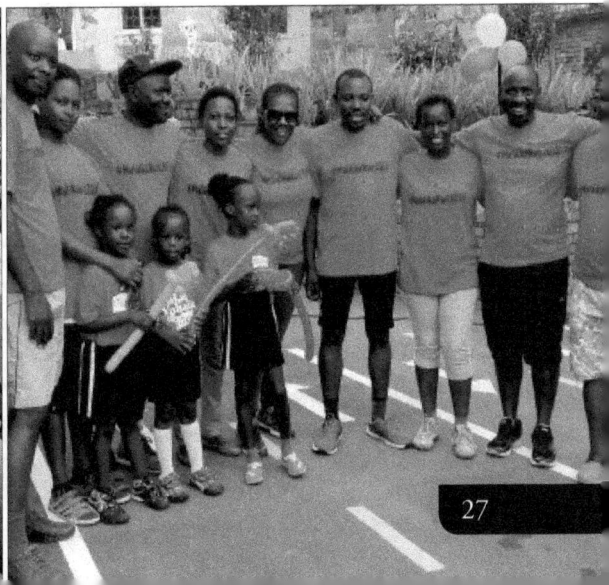

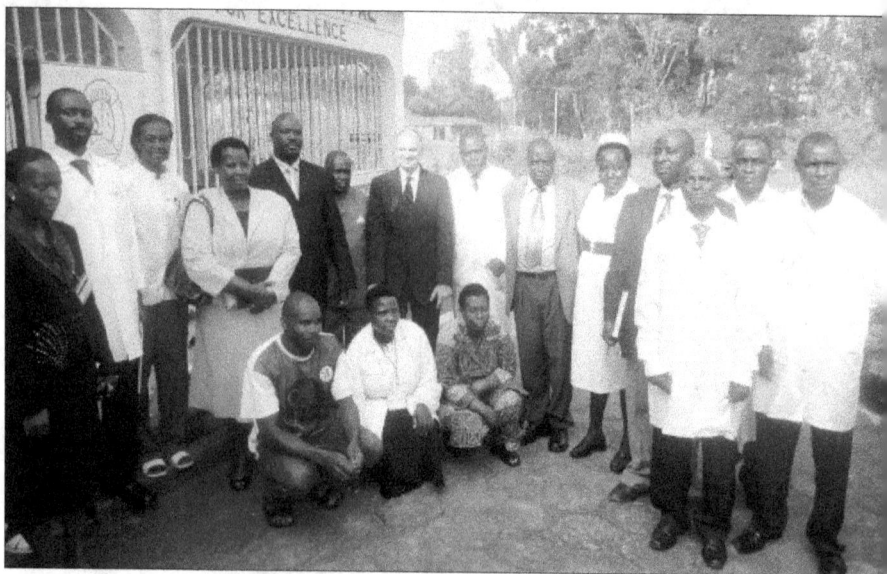

Above: Christine (extreme left) at the visitation of Jerry P. Lanier, the US Ambassador at Fort Portal Regional Referral Hospital and JCRC Fort Portal, 2010. The US through USAID plays a tremendous role in health care and disease control

Below: Christine (fourth from right in orange top) with the Pharma Access (PASER-M) Team at a Resistance network meeting, 2010

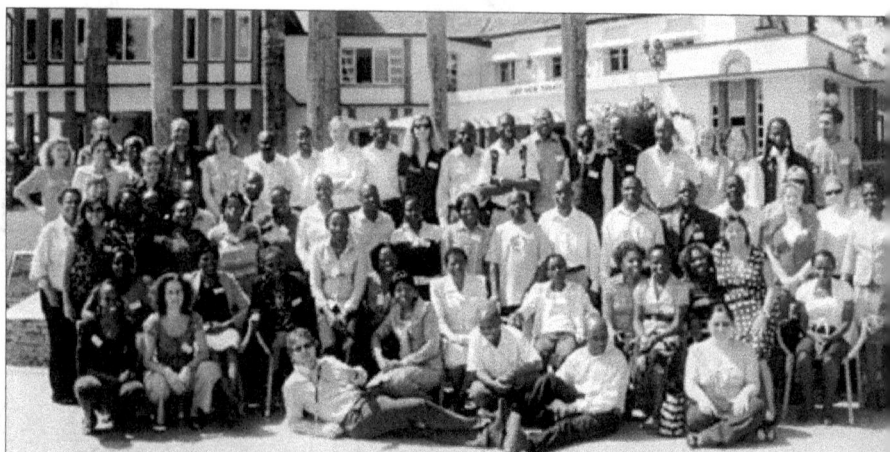

HIV DRUG RESISTANCE NETWORK MEETING AND A.R.T-A WORKSHOP
H-NOV-2010 (ENTEBBE UGANDA)

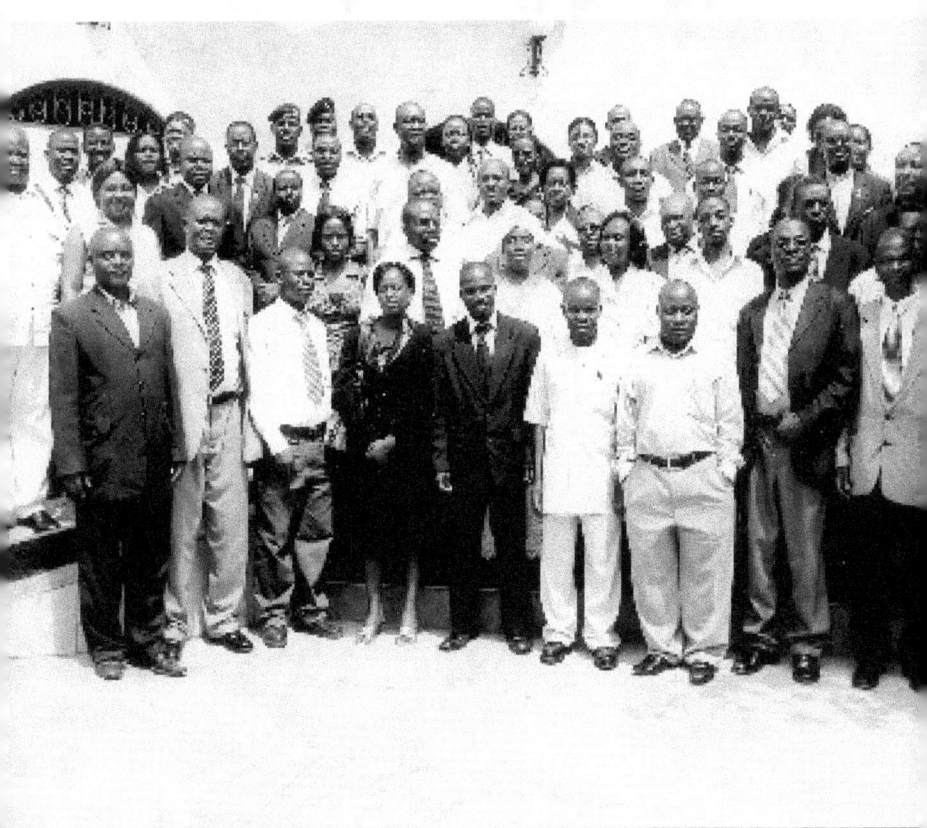

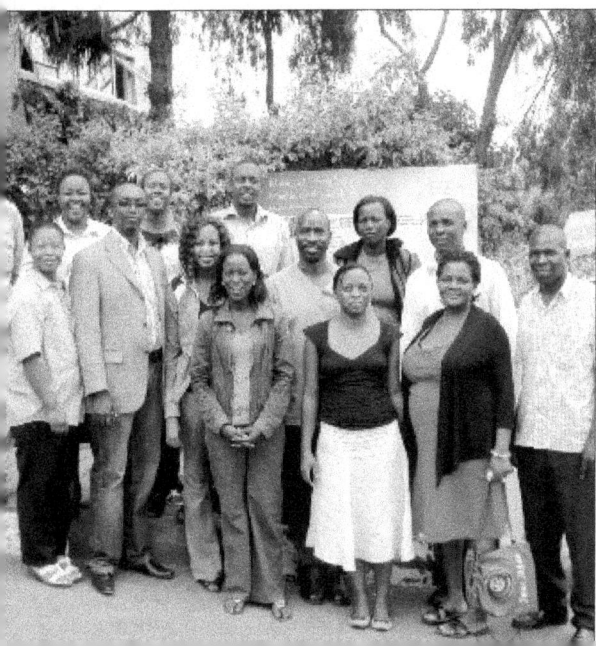

Above: Christine (fourth from left, front row) attending one of the HIV update meetings organised by KAFOFANU, 2011

Below: Christine (fourth from left, front row) and her colleagues (Master of Science in Public Health), 2012

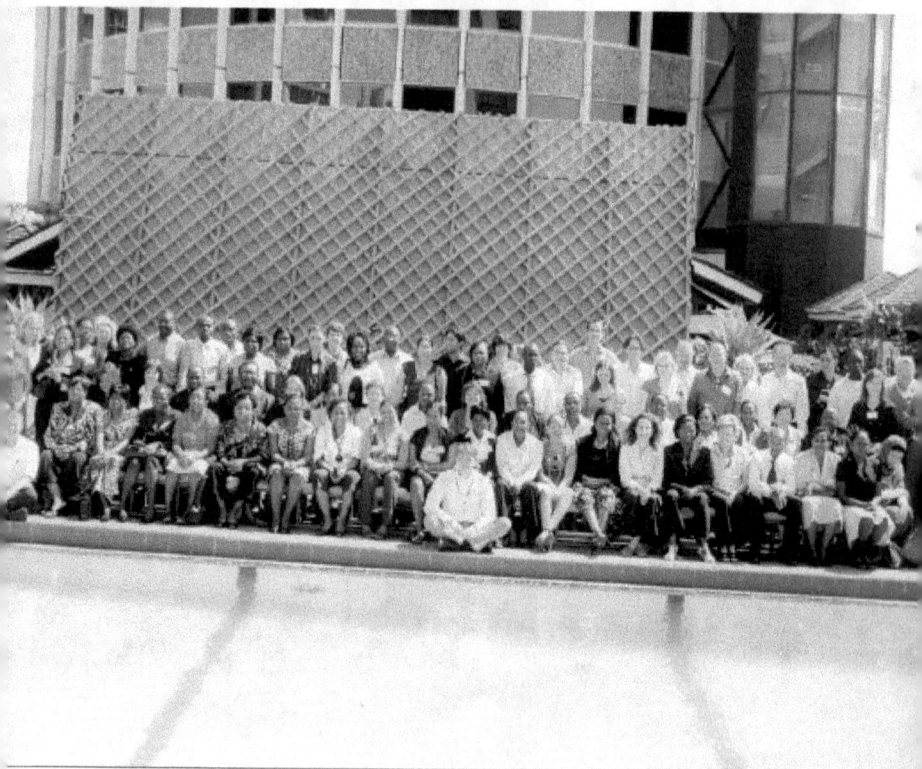

Above: Christine (in the middle row, behind the man who is sitting on the ground) and the Paser-M Team after the network meeting in Nairobi, 2008

Below: Christine (behind the table) and her friends in Nairobi, 2008

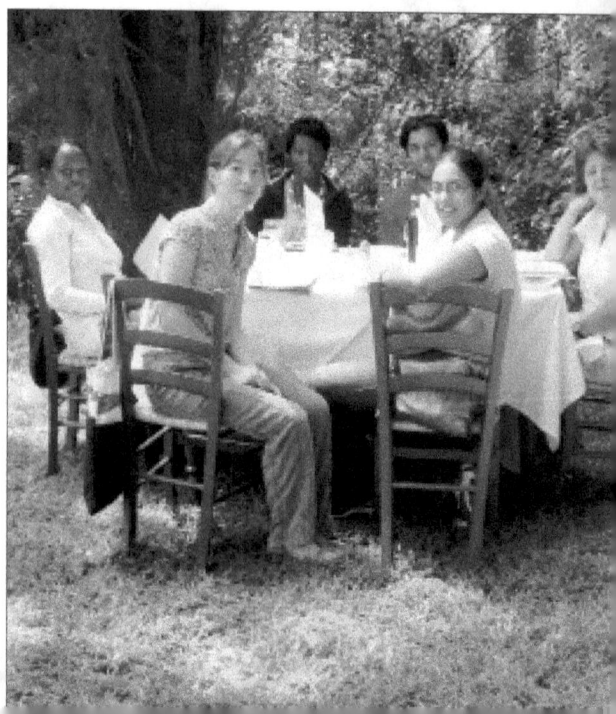

Chapter Three

Chronic illnesses in Africa

Africa faces a burden of chronic and infectious diseases. Many chronic illnesses do not completely heal, and some have no known causative agents. Some are genetically passed on from parents to children and grandchildren. Some are life-long, and people must learn to live with them; eczema is such an example. Other examples of chronic illnesses that can be hereditary include: psoriasis, diabetes and rheumatoid arthritis.

Chronic illnesses are on the increase in Sub-Saharan Africa basically because Africa's health systems, health investments and prioritisation have continued to be inadequate. For example, in Uganda the burden of chronic diseases is generally ignored as can be seen in poor practices and people's poor attitude to seeking health care. One first gets ill in order to seek a doctor's services, this is mainly due to the high cost of consultation services; unavailability of health workers or specialists at health facilities; long distances to the health facilities; ignorance of disease progression; expensive laboratory tests; limited research and pricey drugs. In early 2017, the Food and Drug Administration (FDA) of the United States, approved Dupixent (dupilumab injection) for moderate and severe atopic eczema, but the initial cost is $37,000 per year — making it extremely costly! It is also unavailable in Sub-Saharan Africa.

This has implications for disease control and management. Sometimes people may be lucky to get job opportunities which require that one conducts certain tests before being recruited. These include jobs such as in the military or casual labour overseas. Sometimes schools also require that children/pupils conduct medical examinations before joining a school. This gives such individuals a chance to see a doctor or health worker, an opportunity they would otherwise have not had. If one has not seen a medical practitioner for medical attention, they may have to live with an illness for a long time without knowing it, leading to challenges to disease management and control.

The management of chronic illnesses should take a holistic approach, through advocating proper budgeting and, most importantly, implementing public health interventions to address them. Public health is the art and science of preventing disease, promoting good health and prolonging life through organised efforts and the informed choices of individuals, groups, or organisations. It basically aims at preventing problems from happening or reoccurring.

Focus should be put on effective scientific and preventive interventions like scientific research and collection of information; designing, implementing and evaluating interventions and scaling them in the wider community. Immunisation, for instance, has proved important in protecting people from life-threatening diseases like smallpox, polio, measles and diphtheria. However, weak accountabilities and ineffective systems of monitoring may hinder these developments.

Gaps in the health sector

Uganda's health sector has for many years saved thousands of people's lives. Recently, it was lauded for curbing epidemics, particularly ebola and marburg outbreaks. According to the Ministry of Health 2017 statistics, there are currently 155 hospitals in Uganda. These include two national referral hospitals, 14 regional referral hospitals and 139 general hospitals. Of all these, only 65 are government-aided; 63 are private not-for-profit partnership (PNFP) and 27 are private. This means that most patients have to buy their medications and foot laboratory test costs in the event that they visit non-government hospitals.

There are further gaps in health service delivery, even at the national referral level, including shortage of essential drugs, poorly paid staff, expired drugs, inadequate medical doctors, nutritionists, consultants or expatriates/specialists such as dermatologists. There is also a problem of breakdown of the scarce equipment in the country. The recent breakdown of the only cancer machine which was at Mulago National Referral Hospital is an example. It took almost a year to replace it. In the meantime, scores of patients died and others were flown out of the country to be able to get the services.

Delayed diagnosis

Another major setback in Uganda's health sector is the timing in diagnosis which is partly explained by the scarcity of key staff at health centres. Additionally, there are often variations in the diagnosis made by different personnel on the same patient/ailment. At some point, for example, one doctor will diagnose psoriasis impetigo and the next one will diagnose eczema. It takes a while — even years at times — to make proper diagnosis.

Delayed diagnosis impacts heavily on patients by risking their lives or causing them to incur unnecessarily huge expenses. What is more, owing to the aforementioned lack of equipment in the country, samples may have to be sent abroad for analysis, making the costs even much higher. Delayed diagnosis results in patients presenting with late stages of disease progression.

Unavailability of drugs

There is a shortage of essential drugs at health centres and national referral hospitals to the extent that patients end up buying most of the prescribed medication from private pharmacies owned by business people. This is not only inconvenient, but also costly. WHO (2005) observes that chronic illnesses could cause poverty amongst families and patients.

Limited research and access to information

Research on medical conditions is limited. Health information about several diseases is not available and if it is, it is in medical jargon or even in foreign languages and little information is accessible in the local languages. Even the internet may not be accessible to many due to network problems or affordability. All these factors affect access to vital information.

Competitors — Herbalists

Herbalists have now taken over the work of health centres, meeting patients and prescribing herbs! They go on to educate the patients on herbal medicine as well as exploit chronically ill ones. They have so improved their marketing that they go on television and radio to market their products. This drive by herbalists leads to delayed health-seeking habits; often after herbs fail, patients report to hospitals seeking health care with late stage disease progression, thus making diagnosis and treatment hard. Some herbal medicine may escalate some illnesses and there is not much research to show the interactions of herbals with western medicine. There has been no scientific research follow-up on the use and practices of herbs. There is not even a formal, generic benchmark for addressing quality, quantity and side effects. Herbal concoctions are often not hygienic. One cannot guarantee their shelf life and so they can also be fatal.

Feelings of a chronically ill patient

Accepting the fact that one has a chronic illness may take days. This is mainly because there are a number of things one needs to adjust to, among them the fact that one has to take prescribed drugs for a prolonged period. The following feelings may also occur among the patients of chronic illnesses — as experienced by the author:

Anger

One may feel irritable and anything can make him/her annoyed because of the unpleasant situation he or she is going through. In the case of eczema, reactions develop in uncomfortable places and usually take long to subside. This causes a lot of social discomfort, forcing one to avoid social gatherings. It is important to recognise this and decide not to allow passing thoughts to dictate your present and future because anger cripples love, eats away peace and shatters hope.

Confusion

The situation may be confusing and one may begin to doubt every piece of advice, even from friends. Caution should be taken when communicating information to patients, otherwise, they might be left confused. It is important to support patients to get rid of confusion since it corrodes faith and destroys confidence.

Helplessness

A chronic illiness such as eczema will leave one vulnerable and feeling useless. It can drive you into self pity, and can silence courage. One is left helpless as they see their precious skin, for example, wear away, even when they have seen the best doctors and taken all the medication there is to take.

Fear

Being faced with a life-threatening disease is nothing but a reminder that time is probably up! One is sick, worried and afraid that they will die any time. Worrying and wallowing in despair do not only kill the future, but also ruin the present.

Hurt

Sometimes communicating hurt feelings is not easy, but chronically ill people may be faced with hurt feelings because they are injured and are in agony. The suffering and pain that one is going through is not only distressful but also heart-breaking.

Sadness

Chronic illnesses usually pose a risk of stress and this may leave one sad. Crying spells may be the order of the day due to pain, feelings of shame, or rejection. Unhappiness may be written all over their faces.

Depression

When sad feelings become too much, one's psychological functioning may break down, leading to depression. Sometimes, the re-occurrence of infection is disturbing enough to discourage a patient and send them into depression. At times, the lack of support from a spouse, parents or friends; frequent use of antibiotics and steroids; underlying childhood abuse and too much stress can all result in imbalances in brain chemicals or hormones, leading to depression.

Chronically ill people start to feel they are losing the battle and therefore, have no hope. Depression is not easy to diagnose and may send an individual into neglect, drug abuse and feelings of guilt. They may care less about medicine or food, or grooming. They may experience prolonged sadness, change in sleeping patterns and eating habits, hallucinations, excessive fears and anxieties and constant itching or pain, which affects their mood, and self-esteem. They may even attempt suicide. It is, therefore, important to seek psychiatric attention.

Grief

Grieving is explained by the psychologist Elisabeth Kubler-Ross in her 1969 book, *On Death and Dying*, as a situation when one mourns the loss of anything, including good health or a loved one. When one is bereaved, they may go through the following stages of grief: denial — not accepting that the situation happened; anger — getting angry at the situation or with oneself or with the people around; bargaining — feeling vulnerable and thinking 'if only I had tried to do something earlier'; depression — characterised by total sadness and regret; and acceptance — where the victim comes to terms with the situation.

Indifference

Chronic illnesses can cause one to feel so pathetic that they may start caring less about themselves or others and feel bored.

Medical personnel's mandate

Coping with a chronic illness is not easy as it lasts for a long time and usually with no cure. The emotional dimensions are, sadly, usually ignored by both medical practitioners and caretakers. Management of the illness is usually prescribed through lifestyle changes of diet management, exercise, and some medication.

Clinicians are usually well equipped with skills to help their patients, but often do not know how to deal with the psychological, social and cultural dimensions in health. As such, poor management may affect a patient's ability to cope with medication which can affect treatment outcomes. This calls for a focus on professional development and training to ensure better satisfaction of the patients' needs. A patient may not differentiate between a disease and a disorder. As such, lack of clarity in communicating with a patient may leave him or her perplexed, sad and frightened.

It is important to diagnose and treat psychosocial issues in patients with chronic illnesses to reduce the severity of the condition. The condition provokes feelings of anger, anxiety, stress and depression in extreme cases. These illnesses may also bring about impairment, as in the case of amputation of limbs, loss of vision and so on — making one accumulate fear, and lose strength and focus.

Transmission of stress to the health care workers giving support can only aggravate the situation. This affects performance, so it is important that the health workers become aware of their own mental health to be able to help others.

Side effects and information sharing

All drugs have side effects. Side effects are conditions caused by drugs that one is taking as the drugs take their desired course. These side effects may be minimal, adverse or unpleasant. They range from bad dreams/hallucinations to the development of another illness or bad feelings. Common ones include headache, nausea or vomiting, diarrhoea, poor appetite, dark lines below the eyes, sweating, dryness in certain membranes of the body, excessive sleeping, depression, reduced immunity, and escalation of heart diseases. It is helpful to recognise these and work out a way through them with your doctor because at the end of the day, it helps a patient to understand their medication and facilitate adherence to it.

Having a good doctor-patient rapport is widely encouraged because of the outcomes: it promotes drug adherence and marks the beginning of a healing process. Good rapport can bring about good communication and cooperation between a medical practitioner and a patient, a step necessary for good treatment outcomes. However, at times, medical practitioners do not share information with patients because of the limited time in which they must treat the many others waiting for their service. Some doctors also do not like their patients to make suggestions or advise them, but when there is good communication between the two of you, it is better for patient management, patient understanding and compliance.

Patients who know how to read at times get information from the leaflets inside the packs of drugs while others go on the internet to do some research. As a patient with chronic illnesses, care should be taken to ask about the likely side effects and how to deal with them before you leave the doctor's room. For example, my doctors explained that prolonged use of Prednisolone pills (a type of steroid or corticosteroid) is not good for the immune system and the entire body, yet it works on the immune system itself. This is a drug that seems to work miracles for some patients as it can revert skin reactions within 12 hours of swallowing the first pills, thereby helping the body not to get secondary bacterial or fungal infections.

Steroids or corticosteroids are hormones that are also produced by the adrenal glands which are located above the two kidneys, to prepare the body for fight or flight during stressful conditions. The hormones are responsible for activities like waking up in the morning and other activities including exercise. They also help the body to select the right food nutrients, namely carbohydrates, fats and proteins that the body needs in its physiological activities.

Administration of cortisol drugs helps to regulate inflammation (prevent the release of substances that cause inflammation, rashes, eczema and rheumatoid diseases) and also regulate stress and immune system response. They are different from anabolic steroids that are abused by athletes and body builders to elevate their performance. When using cortisol in chronic illnesses as medication, one needs to be aware of the side effects because of prolonged use. Excessive use of steroids can cause Cushing's or Cushingoid syndrome. It is a disorder that comes because of prolonged exposure of huge amounts of the cortisol hormone to the tissues of the body. It is characterised by an increased amount of fat around the neck, and face.

Steroids are capable of increasing appetite through destruction of the normal metabolic processes. The resulting high calorie intake potentially makes one prone to being overweight. There is also fat redistribution to other parts of the body like the upper arms and stomach; liver and kidney damage; accelerating acne; mood swings; anger; irritability; and thinning of the skin to the extent that bruises occur easily and take longer to heal; weakening of the bones (causing osteoporosis); diabetes and fluid retention in feet; problems with eyes, arteries and blood pressure, including accelerating heart-related complications.

One other side effect that I got from the medication was hypersensitivity of the skin. My skin got super sensitive to almost anything, including hair chemicals. I would also feel overly cold in cold weather. I had the opportunity to discuss with my doctor, how to deal with these side effects of steroids and to find a way forward, as well as agree on which drugs would be suitable for me to take and which ones would not.

For example, I was able to request my doctor not to prescribe Griseofluvin (anti fungal) for me, just before the Government of Uganda stopped its use officially because of its terrible side effects. The side effects were awful; it would cause nausea and vomiting, poor appetite and I would become another kind of patient altogether.

Later I was given Erythromycin (Antibiotic), which was not any different, and yet I had requested my doctor not to prescribe other drugs of the kind including the G.V. Paint 1% (purple liquid) or Coal tar, due to their itching effect.

The other drugs that usually give a hard time are the Doxycyline tabs that have a tendency to cause dark lines below the eyes when one gets exposed to the sun, or generally causing skin pigmentation. When it happened to me, my friends would ask who had given me a hot punch on the face just below the eyes. When I discussed the reaction with the doctor, he advised that I stop taking the drug.

Another sedative drug is Promethazine Hydrochloride. I forgot to ask my doctor about this drug and the next thing that happened to me was excessive sleeping and general body weakness. I would doze off even when I was at work and wondered what was happening to me because I was not under the influence of alcohol and neither did I have sleeping sickness. When I went on the internet and searched for the side effects of the drug, I realised why I was so sleepy!

I then consulted my doctor and he assessed whether it had had its desired effect and he asked me to stop its use, as it was hindering my work and daily life activities. He had to prescribe another drug for me. It is good to search for information on the internet if one has access to it, but in the absence of the Internet, it is advisable to consult your doctor.

The other drug to be aware of is Salbutamol tablets. This is a drug that is prescribed to patients with asthma. I was diagnosed with asthma after prolonged use of steroids. After salbutamol was prescribed for me, it actually worked, because within four days I had improved. The wheezing and coughing which would usually happen at around 3:00am had subsided.

However, I did not have any examinations that were causing me to panic, or hunger and neither was I taking any other medication or alcohol, I started getting tremors or shaking of the hands. Later my legs also started trembling and so I stopped the medication immediately. I consulted my doctor who advised that if the wheezing had stopped, I was free to stop taking the medication as it too was affecting my work and usual activities.

Other side effects of drugs include: generalised body weakness, yellowing of eyes which may indicate other issues such as damage to the liver, frequent thirst, heart complications and diarrhoea.

It is only advisable that one visits a doctor for advice. Some side effects usually do not cause much worry, while others require that one is hydrated all the time, drinking water and juices to help curb the side effects. Some drugs, such as Septrin, cause serious skin burns.

Although drugs may cause such and more side effects, it has been scientifically proven that the advantages of drugs outweigh the side effects. However, the reduction of those side effects goes a long way in providing a good treatment environment for people who have to take drugs for a long time.

Remedial strategies

Personal initiative
Amidst a quagmire of health sector gaps and personal challenges, individual patients can take personal initiatives to ease their respective conditions. This can be done, for example, through making personal observations and risk-free experiments on a diet that suits a health condition. Similar initiatives, such as allowing one space and time for fresh air, sunbathing and spending time in uncrowded places are worthwhile.

Family and friends
In times of need, it is advisable to enlist support from the family. The family offers love, hope, time and their presence is consoling. The family, particularly parents, will tread where most would not dare, even risking their own lives in cases where a condition may be contagious. So, in dealing with chronic illnesses, love is a very important factor for healing. Eating and sharing together, stimulates a lasting bond.

Friends and membership groups, such as faith groups, all make a contribution in alleviating one's adverse health condition.

Such support not only provides confidence but also security, love and care. Besides, such groups often make voluntary financial contributions towards the care of a member or their family. Such gestures taken together with moral support greatly contribute to the healing process.

Facing setbacks

Differences and conflict in family
Due to anxieties and the stress of taking care of a family member with a chronic illness, tensions occasionally build up. People are different and their approaches towards issues differ. At some point the family may get involved in disagreements and a conflict can ensue over issues such as medications suggested by visitors, empathisers and sympathisers. A discussion may result into a quarrel and everyone starts the blame game and squabbling. This has a negative impact on the healing process and may aggravate the situation or, at best, delay recovery.

Finances
Doctors will not tell you this, possibly because they are not financial advisers, but in dealing with a chronic disease money is a big issue. There is a need to have access to money through insurance, savings, investments, or fundraising, in order to access the help that is needed. It is advisable to "make hay while the sun still shines". Encouraging people, especially those dealing with chronic illnesses, to join health insurance, Savings and Credit Cooperatives (SACCOs) is a good idea because it helps them access credit services at a relatively low cost and accessibility is easier than in other financial entities or banks. Savings will help in availing the patient with the basic needs of a balanced diet, decent shelter, appropriate clothing, beddings, and education.

Beneficiaries confess to have been saved by the assumedly little savings that have done wonders for them, especially when they needed to care for the sick and pay hospital bills. When you save with an organised and registered SACCO, the benefits are immense. This is because the group is organised and, therefore, assured of moving forward and developing. It also means there are few conflicts and the dividends are more likely to be high, thus benefiting the members.

Sticking to treatment

Most treatment for chronic illnesses must be taken for life. The majority of these illnesses require drugs and some of these have effects, sometimes fatal, on the body. Although the benefits always outweigh the side effects, it is important to let people know all these obstacles, thus easing the process of adherence to treatment. A lot of well-meaning people in sympathy to the chronically ill, make several suggestions, including deviating from medication and trying other concoctions. However, it is important not to lose focus.

Soothing the effects: Eczema in focus

Taking care of the skin with eczema is a dreaded reality, but bathing with lukewarm water, pat-drying, using a cream to trap moisture, and oiling it with gentle oils can go a long way in providing relief. Olive oil and coconut oil have been recommended because of their anti-inflammatory properties. One needs to avoid using lotions because they get absorbed quickly and one may need to keep applying them. Treatment with topical medicines should be used under the doctor's care or prescription.

Itching, is one of the worst things to deal with as an eczema patient, and is followed by scratching. It is best if scratching is avoided. One can instead apply pressure on the itching parts; keep nails short and wear cotton gloves at night. If the affected area is on the hands, the person can wear disposable gloves. Redirecting one's attention away from the pain and itching by taking a stroll in a cool spot, enjoying the cool breeze from the lake, at the beach or river and travelling to new places is helpful.

Taking advantage of the early morning sun to get Vitamin D or light therapy is another helpful intervention. The doctors recommend at least 10-15 minutes of sun-bathing. Eczema treatment is almost the same for all the types apart from stasis; if one has the stasis type, they should not sit too long and instead try to lose weight and avoid salt or foods that are high in sodium because salt contributes to retaining water in the lower legs and may escalate the problem.

Vitamin supplements may be recommended by the doctors as supplementary, but not as options to medicine. In Uganda our food market is so rich that all our foods are nutritious and supplements may not be required. Avoiding certain foodstuffs like dairy products and peanuts, which are known to cause allergies in some patients, may not be a good idea unless one is sure that indeed it causes them allergic reactions. A balanced diet is an excellent option.

Avoiding the triggers of allergies is key. Efforts should also be made to avoid too hot or too cold temperatures. Avoiding pet fur, cement, sanitisers, wall paint, salon chemicals, food dyes and cloth dyes, dust, smoking, and rough clothing will do the trick. There is also a need to improve one's hygiene such as washing hands often, wearing cotton clothes so that they do not rub the skin, and keeping bathrooms dry and moulds in the interior of the house at bay. Also, be on the lookout for leaking pipes, use unscented products and do away with perfumes. Avoid powder detergents for washing garments because residues of their chemicals remain in the garments and may trigger eczema.

Use fragrance - free products as opposed to unscented products. This is because unscented products may still have some chemical ingredients in different forms and quantities. This means that a masking fragrance may have been added and then you have more chemicals! Most importantly, one needs to avoid stress.

Dealing with self-image

Dealing with self-image, the mind, thoughts and actions is crucial. One who is chronically ill may be constantly engrossed in thoughts and wallow in self pity. One may feel lonely in mind, although he/she may be surrounded by people. The mind is under attack with negative thoughts. Many people will have different conclusions about you; some good and from an informed point of view, others from a position of ignorance. Others will exhibit behaviour that is meant to stigmatise or discriminate against you. In the case of eczema, for example, people will talk about it and refer to it as a skin of a crocodile or a frog, but it is only wise that you do not lose hope.

It is important that you let go of negative thoughts and ignore what other people may think about you and move on positively. One of the avenues to get out of bad thoughts is to engage in outdoor activities like football matches, festival(s), and carnivals. Get involved in adventurous outings, go to the beach, and other similar places. This helps the person to get back on track and maintain a healthy body weight. You must get out of your cocoon and move on.

Telling the tale

Psychologists believe that the more you tell your story the more you are healed from the distresses, thus giving meaning to the old adage, "a problem shared is a problem halved". When told that they have a chronic illness, many people go under cover, calling it a death sentence. Explaining their story over time, makes the story teller feel at ease and, consequently, brings healing while to the listener, it helps them understand and feel comfortable with their condition. This calls for a knowledge upgrade. It is important that the patient gets to know all the information concerning the condition. The patient can keep him/herself abreast of the information from the treating physicians or health workers or surfing the internet.

Chapter Four

Chronic illnesses and supporting others

It is not easy getting a job while one is sick, yet employment is vital and a key source of income because one is able to get funds to buy drugs and for his/her general welfare. It is not easy for employers to employ a sick person, even though Uganda ratified the Employment Fundamental Conventions that protect individuals against labour discrimination. Most people see a sick person as weak and unable to offer services. It may be presumed that the person is falling ill too often and therefore cheating the employer when they take time off work.

One of the ways out of such a situation is volunteering to get and enhance skills that are directly related to one's condition and help them back to normal life. Volunteering is helpful because it is a way of offering a hand of kindness and somehow, benefiting the community as well as getting possible contacts for employment. In a country like Uganda where there are numerous health challenges, as in the case of HIV prevalence, there are opportunities for a chronically ill person to offer help. Specific areas of support include, managing research studies, counselling patients on a whole range of domestic issues such as behaviour change, communication and psycho-social support. While volunteering, it is surprising to see how much patients are capable of sharing, given the chance. People are yearning to share their problems and painful experiences and, in some cases, their knowledge levels are still wanting, especially those from the rural areas. With a caring and supportive person, giving the right information, patients are empowered to deal with their own challenges and conditions.

However, often times, patients battle with disclosure. They wonder how they will communicate the news of a disease or a chronic disorder to their families or friends and how it will be interpreted or perceived. Fear of rejection, stigma and discrimination therefore, needs to be dealt with. Living a sickly life and embracing a disease or disorder takes courage. Bearing the pain, shame, rejection, or even being a laughing stock in the whole village or town is daunting and so one needs proper care and support to be able to cope. Helping patients deal with fear, through education on the condition, sharing the experiences of those with the same condition and empowering them with life skills can go a long way in helping them move on; and because most people, after they have improved, need to be rehabilitated.

Patients struggle, first of all, to deal with the bad or sad news of their diagnosis. In some instances, they struggle to deal with a 'death sentence' as they are told about their condition at health facilities:

> The condition you have is a killer one. You will live with the illness the rest of your life. We have little knowledge on the disease. More research is still going on. The condition you have has no cure. I cannot do much. The medication is not available at the moment. You will swallow drugs for the rest of your life. The clinic has closed; try elsewhere or go and come back tomorrow, etc.

These sound like simple sentences but in actual sense, the patient hearing them is struggling with acceptance. It is not easy, first of all, to accept this kind of communication, let alone deal with it. So, patients need to be helped to understand their condition. They need to be listened to and then allowed to grieve. This is because the condition will have robbed them of their normal life and, therefore, they need some time to "take it in". Some health workers do not have enough time to attend to their many patients; and so, it is a: "come in, get your results, find care in such and such clinic. Next patients, come in!"

Circumstances at their workplaces make some health workers insensitive and depleted of their ability to keep depriving their patients of the opportunity to be helped. Where referral is required, it can save a lot, but it needs to be done in an appropriate manner. The patient should receive an explanation and a proper referral place be identified. A caring health worker may, on an occasion be criticised by workmates for tolerating patients who come late to the clinic, yet asking a patient to go away and come back the following day can be heart breaking. The possible reasons a patient comes late are myriad.

Some patients face a challenge of long distances from their homes to health facilities, where they can see a qualified doctor and have a chance to do a laboratory test and get access to drugs, which are most times unavailable in the clinics near them. Others simply have to depend on others to meet their transport costs and so they have to wait for them to be ready, while for others, it is simply the fact that they are weakened by the illness and require extra time in every preparation they make. Others yet delay to avoid problematic triaging services which are characterised by long queues.

Disease outbreaks and epidemics such as cholera, zika, bird flu, smallpox, plague and ebola impact on patients and health workers. Lack of protective gear, witnessing people dying and others isolated can be nerve-racking and traumatic, bringing disruption in service delivery.

Continuous counselling

Counselling is the continuous process of helping one deal with their problems or challenges. It is not only for the sick. Sometimes, it may include family members and friends through sharing experiences, minimising the annoying effects of the disease, developing plans and the patients deciding on their new choices. It plays a pivotal role in the healing process. A counsellor needs to be up to date with the right information, and thus help people get rid of anxieties as well as provide hope.

Patient associations

In Uganda, little is known about these associations, apart from the Diabetes Association, Sickle Cell Association, Palliative Care Association of Uganda, Association of People Living with Disability, Association of People Living with HIV, Mama Clubs, Down Syndrome Association, Epilepsy Association, Cancer Association, and Uganda Albinos' Association. Other associations for people with disorders and chronic illnesses have not existed or are dormant and not funded. At least I have not heard of one for people with skin disorders.

Associations play a pivotal role in healing since they act as platforms where patients share their experiences and get tips on medication, dealing with side effects and pain management. It is here that dissemination of information happens. In some cases, some members of such associations have found partners from these groups which can be of help and support. A typical picture of positive living can be captured here. We all need social support at some point. These groups play another role of increasing demand for a great deal of services through community engagement to help support rehabilitation services. These play a great role for patients in the terminal phase of their illness.

Modern technology has developed tools to help patients manage triggers, symptoms and share experiences in disease management. For example, the Eczema Association in the United States of America developed an App, My Eczema App, which was designed to give people with eczema and their families a digital platform to track their activities, with the belief that what can be measured can be managed, and all this contributes to research.

Chapter Five

Chronic illnesses in children

Working with children and their caretakers can be a fascinating experience. As adults, we learn a lot from children. Children are told to wash hands before and after eating as well as washing hands after using the toilet to keep germs away. This message sinks in and as grown-ups it goes a long way in improving one's health.

But, children fall sick at times due to their low immunity and innocent exposure to infections while at play, or through their eating habits. They too usually get affected by grief and stress when it comes to illness. They battle with pain and, in some cases, it is hard to understand them until they cry. Children are also infected with chronic illnesses such as asthma, eczema, mental illnesses and permanent injuries that leave them disabled, diabetes, cancers and many others. It is important that we help them understand what is happening to them and empower them to live with these illnesses.

The understanding of chronic illnesses in children basically depends on their level of development, in terms of age and exposure. For example, children below seven years of age may not understand much beyond the simple explanations from adults.

Children need to be given a balanced diet for proper growth, development and cognitive health benefits. It is known that breast milk is the best food a mother can give her baby/toddler because it is whole; it gives the baby all the nutritional values he/she needs. Where babies who are not breastfeed due to elimination of mother-to- child transmissions (EMTCT) or are not responsive to breast milk, more attention may be required including giving fruits and cod-liver oil. Fish can also be given to older children aged 5 to 7 to supplement their nutritional needs.

If a baby does not breastfeed, it may have poor immunity and so nutrition should be considered a priority. Poor nutrition in children leads to stunted growth or failure to thrive. Others, of course, are exposed to infections due to poor immunity, thus exposing them to illnesses. Visiting a nutritionist or a paediatrician for help will also be of benefit to the distressed parent or caretaker.

Schooling

As they grow, it is imperative that children go to school. In some communities, caretakers tend to neglect a child's education when they are battling a chronic illness because they anticipate that they will die anytime, and so "why waste resources!" It is vital for every child to get an education because no one knows when he or she will die. They may actually live to old age with a chronic condition — and many do.

Immunisation

Immunisation should be taken seriously. All children should receive vaccines to build their immunity against deadly diseases. These days, there are a number of programmes to help mothers, which include door-to-door immunisation, child health days, and children's clinic days, where immunisation and shots of vital vitamins are administered. When a child is not immunised, they may suffer from crippling diseases for life or die young. Polio, for instance, can cripple a person for life. It is, therefore, crucial that these health programmes are embraced. It is absurd that due to illiteracy, some sections of society primitively do not believe in immunisation. A multi-sectoral approach to dealing with such issues can be employed and local leaders can help through mobilising communities and sensitising them about the advantages of immunising children.

Disclosure

Some of the knowledge about chronic conditions is associated with superstitions and cultural beliefs, which confuses the children. The reasoning capacity of children improves as they grow. Some children may have heard relatives and friends talk about them and so, they learn from that. The first issue here to deal with is fear of disclosure of conditions such as HIV, considering the stigma that surrounds it. Parents often fear that if they disclose a child's sero-status to them at an early age, the little ones will share the information with the community and put themselves at risk of being stigmatised or discriminated against.

Parents can re-enforce simple pieces of advice such as cleanliness and building communication with the child for future advantage. For children who already have chronic illnesses that have crippled them, it is important that they do minimal exercises at home, like simple games with friends and siblings.

Children above 12 years of age are usually well-informed. Puberty has set in for some, while others have been 'polished' by education. It is through knowing this that we can forge a way of communication to them about their illness and ensure their voices are heard because they also have feelings and many unanswered questions.

Sometimes, disclosure of an illness may happen early or late, depending on the illness. Whatever the case, parents should be consulted by health workers on how to address the issue. At times, the children become suspicious about frequently swallowing drugs even when they are stable. They may also wonder about frequent visits to hospitals, and they try to align what they are experiencing with rumours in the villages or communities. Its important that health workers guide the parents on the process of disclosure. It helps parents create a favourable environment for them to disclose. Children usually prefer getting information from their parents. In the event that they fail, then the health workers can help.

Most health settings have counsellors, psychosocial support staff or social workers who can be of assistance. It is important that confidentiality is kept because some issues such as depression could have been caused by multiple events such as rape or even knowing that they were infected by parents. This requires that these young people be handled with care to instil hope and trust. Many young people battle with abuse and torture, but it is difficult for them to share their pain because they hardly trust anyone.

Matters of sexual health can be addressed here as well. There are many sexually transmitted diseases that can bring a long-term threat to your already chronically ill child. During this stage, many of them are going through body changes and transformation in their sexual parts. A message of prevention of these diseases is vital and extra care for those living with disabilities should be taken.

Parents taking care of chronically ill children need to be encouraged to disclose to at least a few community members who may offer support although some illnesses may come with the risk of discrimination.

Providing role models and allowing the children to mix with their peers helps build their esteem, allows them to get peer support and reduces social boredom. It is important to empower the children to deal with bullying and conflict. Talking or using simple words to explain situations is an ongoing process. In some cases, for example, in HIV cases, health centres, in partnership with the care takers, can facilitate disclosure by supporting parents and asking them questions such as:

- Why do you want to disclose?
- When do you feel comfortable to do it?
- Who would you like to do it?
- How should it be done?
- Who in the family knows or can help, or you would like to also inform?
- How prepared are you for the outcomes
- How will you cope, deal with feelings of anger, fear and so on?

Continuous counselling and education about the condition, while re-assuring the child that having the illness is not the end of the road is key and varies with age. As a child grows, their level of understanding increases and information sharing should be flexible.

Many children regret why their own parents did not disclose the illness to them and yet the parents preferred the health workers to do so. This drives the children crazy and leaves them with mixed feelings. But this is because they fail to understand their own parents' fears and insecurities.

Disclosing plays a vital role in encouraging adherence to medical care — not just drugs but also the instructions that go with them because they will have to take their medication for a long time, or even for life.

Disclosure builds knowledge about the condition; fosters acceptance; helps the child deal with feelings of anger that could result in suicide; and facilitates the learning of coping mechanisms to deal with the illness.

Chapter Six

Taking care of the elderly and those with chronic illnesses

A lot of support is needed for people living with a chronic illness. There are a number of chronic illnesses and conditions that affect the elderly — confusion that affects their emotional health, dementia, cancer of all types, diabetes, hypertension, Alzheimer's disease (forgetfulness), Parkinson's syndrome (which affects the nerves in the brain and the patient presents with tremors), gout, osteoporosis (weak bones), pneumonia, depression, anxiety, heart disease, urinary tract infections, arthritis, and menopause (a gradual and normal condition that all women experience as they age, either just before or after they stop menstruating). Menopause occurs when a woman's estrogenic levels decline, marking the end of her reproductive period, which is usually after the age of 40. Since it is gradual, they may have changes in their monthly cycles, hot flushes, abnormal vaginal bleeding and urinary symptoms, and mood changes or other symptoms, until menstruation ceases for at least 12 months.

Men are affected by andropause. It is a condition that is associated with the decrease in the male hormone (testosterone) as they age. Some experience symptoms that include: fatigue, weakness, depression and sexual problems. They may also be suffering from social issues such as poverty, neglect and death of companions.

The journey of chronic illness is not an easy one. The patient must endure swallowing tablets or insulin needle pricks for life and getting involved in the battle of infection control and management.

The elderly should not be ignored; they need help just like anybody else and their needs are enormous. This is because their aging bodies and reduced immunity make them prone to diseases and illnesses.

Although there has been an evolution in medicine, nothing in this ever-changing world remains constant. More research is still being done to discover the causes and management of these diseases/disorders, and we need to up our game in our struggle; fine-tune our life or at least know what our health is accustomed to.

After knowing how precious our lives are, it is only prudent that we seek to take great care of our lives since we are all candidates for long-term illnesses. Always be on the lookout for warning signs of disease and plan accordingly.

One can get involved in charities to be able to make contributions to support the chronically ill so that they too can live a meaningful life. This practice also goes a long way in mobilising the community and creating awareness of the illnesses. Patient education is vital. It empowers the patients to figure out how to support themselves.

Chapter Seven

Living a healthy lifestyle

When it comes to lifestyle, many think of parties; but it goes beyond that. We want our bodies and mind to be in a great state. There are issues that affect the body, positively or negatively and things we can do or avoid to increase our chances of having good health and a good life. The World Health Organisation (2017) gives tips for a healthy lifestyle, including: eating a healthy diet; being physically active every day; getting vaccinated; doing away with any form of tobacco; avoiding or minimising alcohol; management of stress and having enough rest; maintaining physical and mental health; practising good hygiene; doing away with speeding and drink-driving; using a seatbelt in vehicles; wearing a helmet while cycling; practising safe sex; having regular medical check-ups; and breastfeeding children till the age of 2 years.

Practising good hygiene: techniques of washing hands

Washing hands should be emphasised even in adulthood because it is then that tough and staphylococcus germs or bacteria that cause diseases can be gotten rid of. With clean water and soap, one can get rid of hundreds of germs thereby preventing themselves and others from infections. Get clean water or flowing water and soap, soak both hands and then spread the soap or soapy water all over the hands inside and outside the palms, in between the fingers and the thumb space. Rub thoroughly and then rinse off with clean water. Do this at least before and after eating or handling food, handling patients, using the toilet, or cleaning dirty places. In some cases, a hand sanitiser can be of great help, not withstanding bathing at least twice a day (morning and evening) and wearing clean ironed clothing.

Nutrition and diet

Most of the time, the immune system relies on what we eat. Deficiencies in our diet may manifest in changes in the texture of hair, muscle cramps, numbness in arms or legs and rashes on the face and cheeks. In children, poor diet results in kwashiorkor, rickets, stunted growth or failure to thrive, and beriberi. Today, obesity and anaemia are on the rise as well, in both adults and children, as a result of consuming foodstuffs full of saturated fats, which are not good for the body and deprive it of vital vitamins. This exposes the body to many infections, which the body will not be able to fight off. Scientists have discovered that malnutrition makes people vulnerable to diseases, leading to body malfunction.

People with chronic illnesses need to have a good diet because their immunity needs special attention or to be strengthened to fight off infections. Making the body disease-proof goes a long way. It can be done by consuming foods such as the following:

Low–glycaemic carbohydrates

They are sometimes called energy-giving foods. These are foods that give the body the energy to do daily activities of work and other functions of the body. They include foods such as buck-wheat and wheat products like chapattis, barley, oats, Irish potatoes and, to some extent, the locally grown millet grain in Uganda, which provides iron. Carbohydrate-containing foods are rated on a scale called the glycaemic index (GI). The scale ranks how quickly they increase the glucose or sugar in the blood for a period of about 2 hours when compared with Bread which is placed at 100%. Our entire bodies rely on these sugars to produce energy. The pancreas releases a hormone called insulin, which helps the glucose to move from the blood into the cells. When inside a cell, the glucose is burned along with oxygen to produce energy.

The foods that break down quickly are considered to have a high glycaemic Index (GI) (greater than 70) — for example Cassava, potatoes, Posho, ripe bananas, short-grain rice and white bread. Food with a medium GI (55 to 70) — orange juice, basmati rice, honey, Millet and whole meal bread. Low GI (less than 55) — soy products, milk, pasta, grainy bread, beans, fruits, porridge and lentils.

These will not spike sugar levels in the body. Remember, some medications that people living with chronic illness usually take lead to a high appetite, which is linked to heart problems and makes them prone to diabetes. Foods such as cassava, sweet potatoes, bananas (*matooke*), plantains, and maize meal (*posho*) should be taken in small quantities. Due to their high levels of carbohydrates, one should consider including low glycaemic foods during meals.

Proteins, legumes and seeds
They are at times called body-building foods. Every now and then, the body needs to be repaired and so body-building foods supply the body with rich vitamins such as Biotin (B7) that helps in hair growth, and other vitamins such as A, D, E, and K. Legumes such as peas, groundnuts and deep red beans are rich in fibre. These can

be consumed fresh or dry. Soy-bean is also rich in proteins, but most of what is available on the market is genetically modified and research shows that it is hard to digest in the stomach.

The seeds of pumpkin, flax, sunflower and *chia* have omega-3 and all help in fighting inflammation. All kinds of fish, sea-food such as crabs, lobsters, and star fish, eggs and chicken are other protein-rich foods, but caution should be taken on meat/beef and pork. This is because they contain a lot of fat that could cause obesity. If it must be eaten, it should be roasted first before being cooked. Kidneys are rich in iron and can also be put on your menu.

Healthy fats

They are a rich source of energy and give food flavour. They include: plant oils like vegetable, sunflower, olive, sim-sim, palm, coconut, and avocado oils as well as margarine. Animal sources of fat include cheese, butter, ghee, fish oil and, fatty meat. Care should be taken with regard to the consumption of fats because too much of them can predispose people to obesity and heart diseases.

Vegetables

Greens as they are commonly referred to, play an important role in our bodies. They supply the body with vitamins such as B folate (9), B6, and B12 and minerals. These include, cabbage, cauliflower, broccoli, carrots, bell peppers (green papper, red pepper, and sweet yellow pepper), onions, okra, garlic, and beet root which contain lots of vitamins. There are leafy ones such as spinach (rich in magnesium and potassium), French beans, cassava, and pumpkin leaves, kale (*sukuma wiki*), Amaranth (*Dodo*), and *solanum aethiopicum (nakati)* which is common in all parts of Uganda. Red spinach (*buga*), *Solanum Nigrum* (*nswiga*) from western Uganda, cow peas (*eboo*), and *hibiscus sabdariffa* (*malakwang*) can all be found in Uganda. These provide the body with vitamins A and E, help in blood-formation and are rich in beta-carotenes and antioxidants that are helpful in strengthening the immune system.

Other herbal foods that may be recommended are ginger, cayenne, cumin, turmeric, black pepper, dandelion, cinnamon, and cardamom. They have been advocated by Chinese ancient medicine as foods that boost immunity, encourage weight loss and de-bloating to prevent fat-cell growth and increasing appetite.

Fruits

Fruits are vital in our bodies. One should have at least one fruit serving per day to keep the doctor away. The deep yellow and orange-coloured fruits are richer in minerals, but all fruits provide the body with the necessary vitamins such as vitamins A and C which protect the body against viral infections and inflammation. They also aid in digestion, improve eyesight as well as keeping the bones healthy. They nourish the body and give it energy as well. They include all succulent fruits of tropical Africa and those from abroad. An example of such fruits is pineapples. When craving for sugar, a pineapple is a great substitute. Eating fruits in their raw form helps the body to make use of the soluble fibre (a plant-based nutrient sometimes called roughage which is also a carbohydrate, but does not break down into digestible sugar molecules like other carbohydrates do). The fibre makes one feel full, keeping hunger at bay.

According to the National Institute of Health in the USA, an adult woman needs a 75mg serving of Vitamin C and a male 90mg per day for prescriptions.

Other fruits include: grape fruit, oranges, grapes, passion fruit, sweet bananas, apples, kiwi, lemons, water melons, pawpaw, tomatoes, mangoes, berries, pears, coconut, guavas, bitter melon, and jack fruits. Bitter fruits such as kiwi and bitter melon, are believed to aid in reducing sugar levels in the blood. Bitter melon is better served in cocktail with sweet fruits such as pineapple and passion fruits to improve its taste. If you take the bitter melon and you are diabetic, it is advisable to keep monitoring your blood sugar because it reduces sugar in blood to very low levels.

Some fruits offer an added advantage, since consumption of their roots, stems, leaves and flowers is not only nutritional, but medicinal. For example, pawpaw fruits help in digestion and help fight constipation, but the leaves, when consumed, have anti-cancer components. Mango and orange leaves when consumed or used for a steam bath can help in coughs and colds. Others use fruit leaves, stems and barks for cleansing their skins.

It is advisable to eat the fruits to be sure of a complete serving of fibre and vitamins, although making juice would also be a good alternative. However, when one makes juice from those fruits, they lose the fibre and there is a temptation to add sugar, spiking the blood sugars in one's body.

At times, people choose to detoxify their bodies. Detoxification is the physiological or medical process during which the body eliminates toxic substances in the blood from the liver, through our bowels, the urinary system and the skin. In such cases when they choose to detoxify their bodies, the process is called cosmetic detoxification. They consume only raw vegetables, fruit juice and water for a short period, usually one to five days. This adds antioxidants, vitamins and minerals from raw vegetables and fruits that help prevent or delay cell damage, but it is not completely healthy because it deprives the body of enough energy. This is because one cannot consume fruits and vegetables all the time; the body needs a balanced diet and exercise to be healthy and it will naturally be cleansed.

Milk

Milk is a complete food with essential nutrients for our health. It is rich in calcium that helps in building strong teeth and bones and contains potassium that helps maintain a healthy blood pressure. It also has proteins that help repair muscles and gives energy, although it should be low fat or skimmed and diluted for serving.

Sweeteners

In some cases when a sweetener is required, it helps to consume foods with natural sugar, such as honey, sugarcane, a ripe fruit or sweet potatoes. In case of diabetic patients, caution should be observed and they should have regular blood sugar check-ups.

Flavours

Artificial food flavours are best avoided in case of allergies. Some flavours and spices such as ginger aid in digestion and are also rich in fibre. Natural flavours for beverages should be considered in cases of allergies.

Water

Water is life! An old adage. It should be taken clean and at moderate temperatures. An average person is required to take at least 8 glasses of water — approximately 2 litres — a day. This has far-reaching benefits; to help the body go through its normal metabolism, as the process requires a lot of water. Seventy-five percent of our brains are made of water.

Foods to avoid

There are some bad foodstuffs that we consume on a daily basis just because we do not have time to cook or we are busy at work or on safari.

These foods can easily be accessed in school cafeterias, groceries on road-sides or in trading centres and even in fast-food joints. With all due respect, please do away with processed foods such as cereals and other fortified foods. In studies carried out in the US, they have been discovered to have excessive Vitamin A, Niacin and Zinc. Yes, the body needs vitamins but too much of anything is bad, and too much of Vitamin A, for instance, can result in blindness. It is also linked to liver damage and skeleton abnormalities.

Too much zinc in the body hinders the body from absorbing copper, yet copper is required in the production of red blood cells. This leads to damage of the immune system, which should otherwise be helping to fight off infections. Deep fried foods such as potato chips, plantain chips, banana chips, cheese, salty snacks, crackers, nuts, pancakes, chicken fries, doughnuts, chaps, kebabs, egg rolls and the Ugandan-made pancakes while they are crunchy and appetising delicacies, are also more dangerous than you expect.

They are high in calories and fat which contribute to weight gain and they come in flashy flavours to tantalise you into buying and eating them. They also have a lot of sodium or too much salt, which is linked to hypertension that causes coronary heart disease.

The Ugandan pancake is made of a blend of mashed sweet yellow bananas, cassava flavour, and then cut in a round shape before being deep-fried. People enjoy it and it gives a good serving of reasonable carbohydrates, proteins, natural sugars, fats, vitamin

A, B, C, and minerals. It is a great snack indeed. However, while previously, they would be served hot and fresh, these days, they are packed and in some cases, because of the unavailability of sweet yellow bananas and cassava flour, sugar and maize flour are used as substitutes. Be on the watch for weight gain!

Packed wheat products such as pastries and other carbohydrates such as rice also have a lot of carbohydrates that are associated with weight gain, predisposing one to diabetes and heart diseases.

Packed drinks such as sodas and sweetened juices as well as ice-cream are equally bad. They contain big servings of sugars and artificial sweeteners such as sugar, glucose and dextrose and preservatives such as citric acid, which are linked to diabetes and cancer.

Do away with drinks such as soda and other packed drinks; these not only have a lot of sugar, but also have other hidden properties such as preservatives and citric acid, which play a role in causing havoc to your body. Research shows that with time, these elements turn into carbohydrates and sugar. So, the longer a drink stays on the shelf, the more sugar that forms in it.

Care should also be taken with probiotic products and vitamin supplements. They should be prescribed by a medical practitioner or health worker as deemed necessary. Unfortunately, some companies, in a bid to make abnormal profits, sell to anyone without even assessing their nutritional status. Not everyone needs vitamin supplements all the time and for pregnant mothers, caution is necessary because consumption of too much Vitamin A will be harmful to you and your baby.

Monitoring nutrition

Nutritionists advise that one has to get her weight and height measured periodically as well as a MUAC assessment (Mid-Upper Arm Circumference). This is when a measurement of one's left upper arm is taken using a tape measure designed specially for that, to ascertain their nutritional status. When the measurement is taken and it falls in the green section, it means that the person is well nourished; if it is in yellow, it means they have mild malnutrition and therefore, there is a need to improve. The colour red means that the person is malnourished and may need nutritional supplement and nutrition counselling.

Alternatively, one needs to have their BMI (Body Mass Index) assessed to quantify the amount of mass or muscle, fat and bone a person may have to ascertain whether they have normal weight or are underweight, or overweight. This can be done occasionally. BMI can be calculated by taking one's weight in kilogrammes and dividing it by the height in metres^2 (squared). According to the World Health Organisation (WHO) guidelines, if your BMI is from 18.5 to 25 kg/m^2, this is an indicator of optimal weight. A BMI lower than 18.5 suggests that the person is underweight. A figure from 25 to 30 may indicate the person is overweight. Children and some ethnic groups may not strictly fall into these categories and sometimes males and females differ, but generally speaking, BMI gives a good picture of ones weight status. Therefore, it is necessary to keep one's weight in check in order to prevent chronic illness that come with weight gain or being under weight. The challenge may be in finding a well calibrated weighing scale and a good tape measure to measure height. If possible, seek advice from your doctor.

Food supplements are good and they have played a big role in reducing malnutrition amongst people with chronic illnesses. Food supplements have been 'saviours' to people living with HIV and mostly those with Tuberculosis (TB). TB is a killer bacterial infection that usually infects people with reduced immunity and so people with chronic illnesses can be prone to it. The food supplements on the market or therapeutic foods prescribed nowadays are Plumpy Nut and RUTF. These contain groundnut, milk, vitamins and other minerals. Therefore, if you are already plump, it is best you leave these for those who need them most. It has also come to notice that some people sell them on the streets to people who enjoy delicacies in some cities. The shelf life of these products is compromised since people keep them in unhygienic places and innocent people keep on consuming them, yet these are medical products, which should be prescribed by a practitioner.

Coffee is a fantastic drink right from simply savouring its sweet aroma. It provides a great serving of antioxidants that are an anti-aging component. However, it contains caffeine as well, which stimulates the release of cortisol, a stress hormone, which interferes with the normal metabolism of the body, consequently producing stress. Stress is also linked to heart disease, asthma and the escalation of other immune disorders. So, heavy drinkers of coffee, be on the watch.

Nutrition benefits of different foods and practices

As a patient suffering from chronic illnesses, there is a need to take in the minimum requirement of nutrients to support the body fight infections and to defeat invading pathogens or germs. Long-term illnesses reduce or cripple immunity. There is a need to eat food that will keep the body in shape and sufficiently armoured to fight off infections all the time.

This calls for eating a balanced diet and foods rich in carbohydrates and proteins, fruits, vegetables, some healthy fat and vitamins, all of which can be found in the healthy foods mostly sold in our local groceries. In order for the body to be equipped with the energy it needs, we need to eat and not just eat, but also eat well. Drinking goes hand in hand with this. As the body nourishes itself with food, water, too, is required for better digestion and uptake of nutrients for use in the body.

Surprising effects of fasting

Today it has become a norm for people to fast, with people going without food for an entire day or going without specific foods for specific periods mainly for religious or health reasons. It is not healthy for one to do without food for a long period, but there are some benefits if fasting is done intermittently or from time to time. When we fast, our bodies get restricted in the uptake of calories, consequently improving our general health. Fasting also facilitates the use of fat stores and glucose to produce energy, lowering the metabolism rate and the blood pressure.

Fasting helps the obese to cut down on weight and promotes detoxification since toxins are stored in fat. When the fat is broken down to give you energy, the body gets cleaned up. However, not all chronically ill people need to fast and when breaking the fast, it is prudent to have a balanced diet, starting with soft foods. Our bodies are massive engines, just like the engine of the car and they need servicing — the service is food.

Importance of sleep

Sleep is an important factor in life because it allows the body and mind to rest and then one wakes up fresh for another day. As a person living with a long-term illness, there is a need to get adequate sleep. Sleep is composed of REM and Non-REM. REM means Rapid Eye Movement sleep while Non-REM means Non-Rapid Eye Movement sleep. Lots of dreams happen during REM.

A lot of people deprive themselves of sleep in a bid to work hard and at times, others deprive themselves of sleep while they are having fun and going on drinking sprees. Some medications and diseases cause insomnia (lack of sleep). Research shows that one needs to sleep at least 8 hours a day. It is important to go to bed early and wake up early. Like the saying goes: "Early to bed and early to rise, makes a man healthy, wealthy and wise".

Lack of enough sleep, especially in the morning, can cause obesity and fatigue. It is also linked to intestinal diseases, cardiovascular diseases and aging.

Sometimes people experience sleep disorders such as insomnia, where one fails to sleep. This is evident among chronically ill patients. Eczema patients, for instance, find it hard to sleep because of their itchy body/skin.

To have a great night's sleep is to ensure that one exercises regularly; has a shower just before bed; reads an exciting book before bed; or watches an exciting film/video. Ensure that your bedroom is clean, quiet, cool and dark. Always associate bed with sleep. Lie down when you mean to sleep. Ensure that you are not taking alcohol or smoking.

In less serious cases of insomnia, a deep breathing exercise can help. Lie down relaxed on your back with arms straight close to your body. Close your eyes. Take in a deep breath then breathe in and out for 5 seconds and sleep should come in a few minutes. This is because the brain gets supplied with plenty of oxygen, consequently inducing sleep. Also ensure a sleep rhythm by sleeping and waking at the same time everyday so that the body learns to control itself. This should help people experiencing insomnia and those experiencing itching or pain.

Another sleep disorder is snoring. One has to observe how they sleep. Sometimes, there may be a need to change the position of the head of a snoring patient a little, to reduce the snoring. Ensure that the head is resting well on the pillow or bed and is not sharply bent.

The other sleep disorder that people living with chronic illnesses may encounter is sleep-walking. Some people may act out their dreams, talk, scream, punch, kick and even walk as if they are awake yet they are deeply asleep. It is important that family members are aware of this and always help redirect the patient back to bed in a calm manner.

The other disorder is hallucinations. These could be linked to some drugs. It is important to recognise the cause and work with your doctor to work out a way through them. Drug induced hallucinations subside as one gets accustomed to the drugs, usually this takes about 2 weeks. A case in point is people on psychiatric medicines or antiretroviral drugs (ARVs) such as Efavirenz.

Dreams are generally a way the mind tries to empty the repository of information to make way for new information the following day and in so doing, the brain taps in the unconscious, as Carl Jung, a great psychologist, states. According to Pamela Ball in her book, *10,000 Dreams Interpreted*, dreams serve two purposes: one is correct sorting and filing of information; and two is the presentation of information necessary for the dreamer to function successfully within the world. She asserts that interpretation of these dreams requires that they are interpreted from more than one perspective in order to be able to fully understand them; including the science of the dreamer's understanding.

Restraining from drug abuse

What are drugs and what are they capable of inflicting on a chronically ill person? These are substances in the form of liquid, plants or synthetic material which when taken by a living organism, modify their functionality. Examples of substances or drugs abused include: nicotine and narcotic drugs such as khat, marijuana, cocaine, heroin, and inhalants such as aerosol and alcohol. They can increase the rate or intensity of one's mental and physical activity like hypnosedatives, which are actually drugs that are given to mental health patients. They get abused because of their ability to make someone calm and relaxed. Hypnosedative drugs should only be prescribed and monitored by medical practitioners.

Chronically ill people should also be careful about alcohol as it can aggravate the problem. Patients with a mental health disorder should be particularly careful.

Alcohol moves from the mouth to the stomach, and then to the circulatory system, brain, kidneys, lungs and liver. Patients with a mental health disorder must take extra precaution on this.

It is responsible for most mouth and throat cancers, and it damages the liver. Since it is in form of small molecules, it is wholly absorbed in the stomach and blood stream. It dilates or widens the vessels, leading to flow of blood to the skin and contributes to a drop in blood pressure. In the end, it affects the body's ability to control behaviour and body functions.

Abusing drugs has partly been responsible for family breakdowns, yet families are support centres for patients. Drug abuse is also responsible for increasing health problems and mental disorders, sexual promiscuity and illicit demand for drugs.

People battling chronic illnesses should restrain from these as they impact negatively on their already weak immune systems and accelerate the severity of the long-term illnesses.

Resisting drugs at times may be hard, especially when it is driven by peers or if there is addiction. But it is only wise to seek help from responsible people or health facilities. The first step towards getting rid of drugs is to recognise that they are not good, but trying to replace a bad habit with a good habit. For example when smokers have the urge to smoke, they can instead make their mouth busy with sugar free chewing gum. If one drinks alcohol, he/she may reduce their intake gradually, from 20 bottles to for example 10 and then 5. One can keep reducing till they never need to take alcohol and when they feel the urge to drink, they can drink other fluids like juice and tea. Remember, alcohol and drugs not only compromise mental and physical health, but are responsible for damaging work and family life.

Avoiding stress

Stress is a response by one's body to protect them from danger or pressure. What may be stressful to one, may not be so, to another, so stress varies from individual to individual. It can also be difficult to measure. When the body is confronted with external pressure, in response, the brain stimulates the production of a hormone called cortisol which can trigger cravings for sugar and fat. This can be detrimental when it comes to long-term illnesses as it can cause obesity.

Stress also contributes to headaches, interferes with memory, work, sex drive, accelerates skin disorders such as acne and psoriasis, and leads to chronic pain and faster ageing. When it is not managed well, stress can lead to depression.

Stress is capable, therefore, of accelerating any illness irrespective of the care. Avoiding seemingly trivial situations may be essential. These may include things such as traffic jam, rush hours, as well as stress from friends and work situations. Incorporating stress management techniques in one's daily life can help one deal with many issues.

Avoiding stress at work
At a work place, it easy to get stressed by many issues, ranging from individual to managerial or institutional.

Individual sauces of stress
On an individual level, one may be struggling with too much work, failure to complete work on time and backlogs; late coming; poor time management; rush hour or traffic jam; and the indiscipline of co-workers, causing conflict and introducing politics and faith issues at work. It is important to keep time and plan one's work appropriately. It is important not be over-sensitive to negative critics but rather pay attention to the mistakes and get them corrected. Above all ensure good communication practices.

The institution as a source of stress
The institution or work place can be a source of stress. For instance, when systems are not in place or are down, conflicts may arise among staff. Systems include working procedures or policies. The absence of human resource manuals can result in stressful situations. Poor or inadequate safety measures and lack of job descriptions can be a source of stress because staff will be caught

off guard and clash in their roles, while poor safety policies lead to deaths or serious illnesses.

Bad managers as stressors

According to Vicky Oliver in her book, *Bad bosses, crazy co-workers and other office idiots*, a few traits of supervisors and other co-workers may have a negative effect on you. Here is how to identify a bad manager who may be a source of stress. Bad managers think that they are right all the time. How possible that is, I will not be able to tell you! They expect you to just be like them. They always change their mind. They never give you feedback; they think it is not important for you to get feedback from them usually because they are hiding something from you. This will eventually cause a lot of discomfort and frustration and consequently stress you at work because you are working hard to please and avoid embarrassment.

They never show any form of appreciation for the work that you do, but will blame you for all the mistakes, usually publicly and yet they take all the credit as if you were not part of it. They come up with work for you during your free time or preoccupy you, making work your identity. If you are battling a chronic illness, and you consider how many hours you must spend with this person in a day or year, you may start having sleepless nights, consequently getting stressed. Your family will also be affected. Prof. Ferguson, an assistant Professor at Utah University, in studies he co-authored which were conducted at Baylor University in the USA, called it a spill over effect, where your working condition affects your relationships, health and other areas of life.

What should be clear is that you do not owe your health to your boss and neither should you compromise your family because of work! It is only wise that you treat others with respect; keep your documentation proper; try and be peaceable with everyone (although your rationality must be known); treat hurt feelings with respect; set a reasonable standard of conduct and in extreme cases, please seek help from resourceful people.

Exercises for Chronic Illness

Exercises for a chronically ill patient

People with chronic illnesses need exercise, just like any other individual, for fitness. Secondly, because they are usually on medication, some of which brings about obesity, exercise for example, walking, running, yoga, swimming, aerobics, dancing, hiking, house work and gardening comes in handy.

Sitting for long hours affects the body's metabolic activity. The body needs to exercise so that it can use the sugar in the body or break down carbohydrates to be able to generate energy for us. If not broken down due to a sedentary lifestyle or sitting for a long time, the carbohydrates are converted into sugars and the results will be disastrous. The body needs exercise for at least 30 minutes every day. These days, people's sitting postures are also destructive; one sits leaning forward while bending their back sharply.

This breaks the spine and when coupled with lack of exercise, results in the development of sedentary lifestyle illnesses such as diabetes and spinal injuries. The right way to sit is upright with the back of the chair supporting your back. It is advisable that one leaves their seat every two hours to stretch. Avoid having your lunch from the same seat from which you work. Some exercises that can be performed at work, right at your desk, include:

- Sit straight, unfold your arms and legs, then stretch your arms up in the air and stretching your legs far forward while seated, take 10 deep breaths and then pull your legs back. Do this at least two times.
- Try to sit on a chair that has a cushion that is straight to support your back. Leave your seat and make short movements after every two hours.
- Stretch your left arm over your head and try to reach your right arm until you feel the tension as you stretch. Let your elbow touch your head from behind. Hold your arm for at least one minute and then change to the other arm.
- Twist the head side ways from left to right.
- Stretch your hands and try to reach your toes.

Another good exercise is walking. There are however some dos and don'ts of walking. Set your mind to it and then get the right attire (light clothes and good canvas shoes or flat shoes). Do not over-stride to elongate your steps, rather take quick and short strides. Walk upright, head parallel to the ground and swing your arms from the front to back with elbows close to the body. Avoid swinging your arms sideways. Avoid landing the entire foot on the ground, rather aim at rolling forward. And, of course, avoid carrying heavy items.

Relaxation exercises

Since we spend most of our time at work, it is important to try out the exercises that I have already talked about above to help relax the body. These include walking, stretching while you sit, and running.

It is important to identify stressors and eliminate or avoid them.

Under stressful or difficult situations which include times of illnesses, one may perform a simple but helpful relaxation exercise like yoga. It helps put the mind on some sort of holiday. Avoiding distraction; get away from the phone and computer. Remind yourself of your successes no matter the years back. Success is success!

Start by tidying yourself up and then find a quiet and comfortable place. Remove unnecessary clothing. Sit comfortably. Close your eyes. Think of the best place you have ever visited. Think of yourself wearing your best clothing and ready to go to that place. See the nice colours around, smell scent of freshly blossoming flowers and feel the cool breeze from the ocean or lake. Forget the money issues and the haters. Be happy. Imagine you are there; you have just arrived. Relax your muscles. Relax your head, neck, jaws and shoulder muscles, and the rest of the body.

Bibliography

Ama de-Graft Aikins. Tackling Africa's chronic disease burden: from the Local to Global. .BMC. Available at: https://globalizationandhealth.biomedcentral.com/ articles/10.1186/1744-8603-6-5 -- Accessed 4th October 2016

America Academy of Dermatology/Association. Scalp psoriasis. Available at: http://www.aad.org/skin-conditions/dermatology-a-to-z/scalp-psoriasis/ Accessed 2016

Anderson, P. & Baumberg, B. (2006) Alcohol in Europe, A Public Health Perspective. A Report for the European Commission. London: Institute of Alcohol Studies.

Atopic Dermatitis. Available at: www.medicinenet.com/atopic_dermatitis/article.htm

Ball, P. (1996) *10,000 Dreams Interpreted*. Leicester, UK: Arcturus Publishing Ltd.

Boston, Gariella. Prediabetes doesn't have to be a 'doom's day message': what you need to know, and do. Washington post. Available at: https://www.washingtonpost.com/ lifestyle/wellness/prediabetes-what-you-need-to-know-and-do/2016/10/18/980fe614-90ad-11e6-a6a3-d50061aa9fae_story. html

Charlotte LoBuono For the first time, study proves Eczema is an autoimmune Disease. Health Line. Available at: www.healthline. com/healthnew/stach. Acessed October 2016

Cunliffe, Tim Seborrhoeic-eczema . The Primary Care Dermatology Society. Available at: http://www.pcds.org.uk/clinical-guidance/seborrhoeic-eczema Accessed 16 July 2016

Eczema: Light therapy and oral medications. Available at https://www.ncbi.nlm.nih.gov/pubmedhealth/PMH0091221/ Accessed 23, February 23, 2017

Five not possible things you can do to make yourself healthier Published by Yahoo lifestyle Available at: https://www.yahoo.com/beauty/5-things-know-trying-elimination-220745319.html Accessed in October, 2016

http://www.cheatsheet.com/gear-style/sensitive-skin-products-you-shouldnt-use.html/?a=viewall Accessed November, 2016

http://www.mayoclinic.org/diseases-conditions/psoriasis/basics/definition/con-20030838 Accessed in June, 2015

http://www.statehouse.go.ug/media/news/2014/06/12/ budget-speech-financial-year-201415-delivered-meeting-4th-session-9th-parliament Accessed 14 April, 2018)

https://www.yahoo.com/beauty/39-healthy-39-is-in-the-body-1536529808588854.html Accessed in October, 2016

Illness and healing. Journeyanswers.com Available at: https://journeyanswers.com/illness?nPartner=enAdwords10&gclid=CLDX2u6G588CFQ88GwodFToNSA Accessed in October, 2016

Website (2017) Food and Drug Administration (FDA). https://www.fda.gov/newsevents/newsroom/pressannouncements/ucm549078.htm

Website Ministry of health http://health.go.ug/affiliated-institutions/hospitals Accessed 14th July 2017

Institute for Quality and Efficiency in Health Care, 2017 February, 23. Eczema: Light therapy and oral medications . Pub Med Health. Accessed 23 February 2017

Jenifer D. Hamilton et al. 2014, December. Dupilumab improves the molecular signature in skin of patients with moderate-to-severe atopic dermatitis. *Journal of Allergy and Clinical* immunology Available at ttps://www.sciencedirect.com/science/article/pii/S0091674914014833 accessed 2017

Jennie Wright-Paker website, 7 stages of Grief-recover from Grief. Recover-from-grief.com Available at http://www.recover-from-grief.com/7-stages-of-grief.html Accessed January, 2017

Jess Bolluyt.7 ways you should switch up your skin care routine for fall Published by Cheat sheet http://www.cheatsheet.com/gear-style/switch-skincare-routine-fall.html/?a=viewall Accessed November, 2016

Julie Axelrod. The 5 stages of grief and loss. Central Com   Available at http://psychcentral.com/lib/the-5-stages-of-loss-and-grief/accessed 2018

Kay Shou-Mei Kane et al. (2002) Eczema Health Centre, 8 Types of Eczema. Web MD. Ministry of health http://health.go.ug/affiliated-institutions/hospitals http://www.webmd.boots.com/skin-problems-and-treatments/eczema/eczema-types Accessed on 29 May 2017

Korin Mille. 6 nutrients you should be eating for healthier hair. Available at: https://www.self.com/story/6-nutrients-you-should-be-eating-for-healthier-hair Accessed October, 2016

Kubler-Ross, Elisabeth (1969) On *Death and Dying*. New York: Macmillan.

Kübler-Ross, Model. Feeling white: Whiteness, emotionally and education. Available at: Wikipedia https://en.wikipedia.org/wiki/K%C3%BCbler-Ross_model Accessed January, 2017

Lauren Weiler. These fruits are even healthier than you think. Cheat Sheet. Available at: http://www.cheatsheet.com/health-fitness/

fruits-healthier-than-you-think.html/?ref=YF&yptr=yahoo
Accessed 16 December 2017

Lauren Weiler. 6 Tips to help you get rid of belly fat- seriously. Cheat
Sheet. Available at: http://www.cheatsheet.com/life/tips-get-rid-of-
belly-fat.html/?a=viewall Accessed October, 2016

Maia. 18 important nutrients you've never heard of—and where to
get them. reb book. Available at:https://www.redbookmag.com/
body/healthy-eating/g3808/lesser-known-nutrients-your-body-
needs/?slide=1 Accessed October, 2016

Marrisa Oliva. 4 things to do right now for younger looking skin. red
book Available at: https://www.yahoo.com/beauty/4-things-now-
younger-looking-162126457.html Accessed October, 2016

Mary Kiconco Begumya-Ogara, M. (2015) *One hundred Locks, insights
for the Christian Single*. Bloomington, Indiana: WestBowPress.

Mayo Clinic Web site. Psoriasis-Symptoms and causes. Available at:
www.mayoclinic.org/disease-condition/Asia/ba

Ministry of Health, National Health Policy and strategic plan
for Cayman Islands 2012-2017 Available at: http://www.
ministryofhealth.gov.ky/sites/default/files/MHEYSC_
NATIONAL_HEALTH_POLICY.pdf Accessed 14 July 2017

Morin , Amy. 7 Ways to Heal Your Body by Using the Power of Your
Mind, Backed by Science. The Inc life. Available at: https://
www.inc.com/amy-morin/7-ways-to-heal-your-body-by-using-
the-power-of-your-mind-backed-by-science.html Accessed 24
October 2016

Mugyenyi, P. (2012) A *Cure Too Far: the Struggle to End HIV/AIDS*
.Kampala: Fountain Publishers.

National Eczema Association. Eczema Lifestyle. Available at: https://
nationaleczema.org/eczema/lifestyle/

Oliver, V. (2008) *Bad bosses, crazy co-workers and other office idiots.* Naperville, Illinois: Sourcebooks.

Pub Med website. Eczema: Light therapy and oral medications. Available at: https://www.ncbi.nlm.nih.gov/pubmedhealth/ PMH0091221/ Accessed February 23, 2017

Republic of Uganda, Ministry of Health (2010) *Integrated Management of Acute Malnutrition Guidelines.* Kampala: Ministry of Health.

Sam Becker, Sam. The Best exercises to boost your metabolism. Cheat Sheet. Available at: https://www.cheatsheet.com/health-fitness/ exercises-that-will-boost-your-metabolism.html/?a=viewall Accessed October, 2016

Speech, Financial Year 2014/15 Delivered at the Meeting of the 4th Session of The 9th Parliament of Uganda on Thursday, 12th June, 2014 by Honourable Maria Kiwanuka Minister of Finance, Planning and Economic Development Available at: financial year report 2014/2015

Taryn Brooke. Sensitive skin? 4 Skin products you should never use. Cheat Sheet Available at: http://www.cheatsheet.com/gear-style/sensitive-skin-products-you-shouldnt-use.html/?a=viewall Accessed November 26, 2017

The Good News Bible (1976) New York: Bible Societies, HarperCollins.

The Mighty, October, 'Healthy' Is in the Body of the Beholder. Yahoo life style. Available at: http://www.yahoo.com/beauty/za

Turner, Jane and Kelly, Brian. Emotional dimensions of chronic disease. PMC. Available at: https://www.ncbi.nlm.nih.gov/pmc/ articles/PMC1070773/ Accessed October, 2016)

UNAIDS (2006) Global AIDS Epidemic Report . Geneva, Switzerland.

Web MD. Skin problems and treatment Guide Available at: http:// www.webmd.com/skin-problems-and-

Weird signs you're vitamin deficient. Fox News Health. Available at: http://www.foxnews.com/health/2016/03/24/5-weird-signs-youre-vitamin-deficient.html?utm_source=zergnet.com&utm_medium=referral&utm_campaign=zergnet_1073474 Accessed October, 2016

Zijlstra , E.E. and Alva, J. (Eds.) (2004) *The Clinical Book.* 2nd Edition, 2008. Department of Medicine, College of Medicine, Malawi.

Index

www.ingramcontent.com/pod-product-compliance
Lightning Source LLC
Chambersburg PA
CBHW052013270326
41929CB00015B/2906

Heroic Struggle: Coping with Chronic Illnesses
— Personal Eczema Experiences